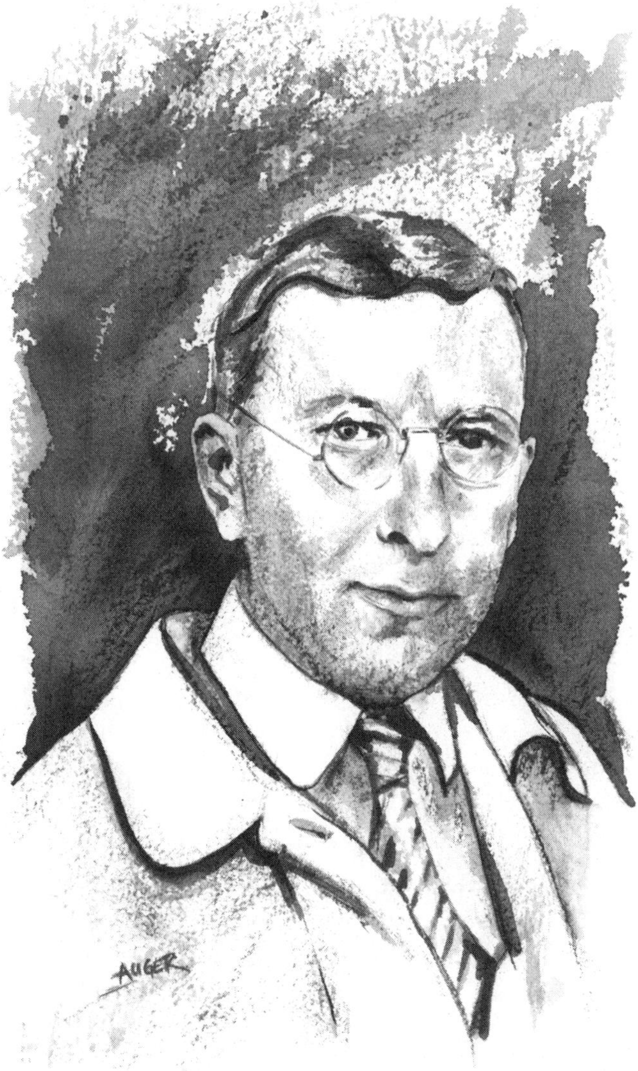

Frederick Banting, 1891-1941.

Artist: Francine Auger

Stephen Eaton Hume

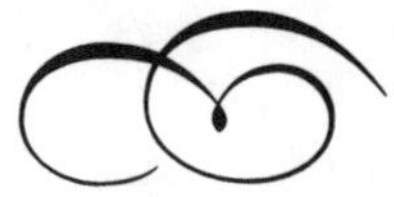

Stephen Eaton Hume was born in Dallas, Texas. He grew up in Texas, Hawaii, and southern Maryland, and spent the summer holidays at his grandfather's home overlooking the water in Upper Blandford, Nova Scotia. He attended Trinity College in Hartford, Connecticut, and the University of Toronto. He now lives in Victoria, B.C. and teaches at the University of Victoria.

He has written three picture books – *Midnight on the Farm*, *Rainbow Bay*, and *Red Moon Follows Truck* – as well as a young-adult novel, *A Miracle for Maggie*, which tells the story of a brave young girl and her battle with diabetes. Stephen Eaton Hume is also an award-winning journalist, and his articles on health care, media ethics, and other subjects have appeared in *The Journal of the American Medical Association*, *The Globe and Mail*, and *The Medical Post*.

THE QUEST LIBRARY
is edited by
Rhonda Bailey

Editorial correspondence:
Rhonda Bailey, Editorial Director
XYZ Publishing
P.O. Box 250
Lantzville BC
V0R 2H0
E-mail: xyzed@telus.net

In the same collection

Ven Begamudré, *Isaac Brock: Larger Than Life.*
Lynne Bowen, *Robert Dunsmuir: Laird of the Mines.*
Kate Braid, *Emily Carr: Rebel Artist.*
William Chalmers, *George Mercer Dawson: Geologist, Scientist, Explorer.*
Betty Keller, *Pauline Johnson: First Aboriginal Voice of Canada.*
Dave Margoshes, *Tommy Douglas: Building the New Society.*
Raymond Plante, *Jacques Plante: Behind the Mask.*
Arthur Slade, *John Diefenbaker. An Appointment with Destiny.*
John Wilson, *John Franklin: Traveller on Undiscovered Seas.*
John Wilson, *Norman Bethune: A Life of Passionate Conviction.*
Rachel Wyatt, *Agnes Macphail: Champion of the Underdog.*

Frederick Banting

Canadian Cataloguing in Publication Data

Hume, Stephen

Frederick Banting: hero, healer, artist

(The Quest Library ; 12).
Includes bibliographical references and index.

ISBN 0-9688166-3-0

1. Banting, F. G. (Frederick Grant), Sir, 1891-1941. 2. Diabetes – Research. 3. Physicians – Canada – Biography. I. Title. II. Series: Quest library; 12.

R464.B3H85 2001 610'.092 C2001-940385-2

Legal Deposit: Second quarter 2001
National Library of Canada
Bibliothèque nationale du Québec

XYZ Publishing acknowledges the support of The Quest Library project by the Canadian Studies Program and the Book Publishing Industry Development Program (BPIDP) of the Department of Canadian Heritage. The opinions expressed do not necessarily reflect the views of the Government of Canada.

The publishers further acknowledge the financial support our publishing program receives from The Canada Council for the Arts, the ministère de la Culture et des Communications du Québec, and the Société de développement des entreprises culturelles.

Chronology and Index: Lynne Bowen
Layout: Édiscript enr.
Cover design: Zirval Design
Cover illustration: Francine Auger
Photo research: Cynthia Cecil

Printed and bound in Canada

XYZ Publishing
1781 Saint Hubert Street
Montreal, Quebec H2L 3Z1
Tel: (514) 525-2170
Fax: (514) 525-7537
E-mail: xyzed@mlink.net
Web site: www.xyzedit.com

Distributed by:
General Distribution Services
325 Humber College Boulevard
Toronto, Ontario M9W 7C3
Tel: (416) 213-1919
Fax: (416) 213-1917
E-mail: cservice@genpub.com

STEPHEN EATON HUME

Frederick BANTING

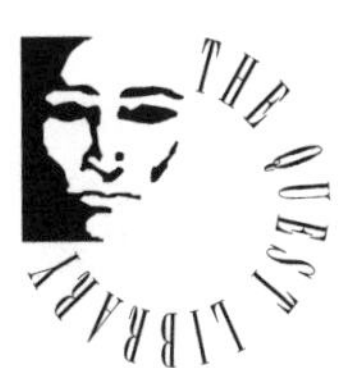

HERO, HEALER, ARTIST

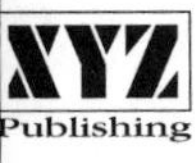

Acknowledgments

I would like to thank my editor Rhonda Bailey; Cynthia Cecil, who researched photos and paintings; Kitty Lewis for her research at Banting House in London; Jennifer Lee, diabetes educator at the Royal Jubilee Hospital in Victoria, for reading the manuscript; Henri Wetselaar and Scott Munro of the Greater Victoria Public Library for showing me rare copies of *The Pilgrim's Progress* and A.Y. Jackson's book, *Banting As An Artist*; and the staff members of the McPherson Library at the University of Victoria for their help and support.

He turneth the wilderness into a standing water, and dry ground into waterprings. – Psalm 107: 35

This book is for Jack and Dianne Hodgins

Contents

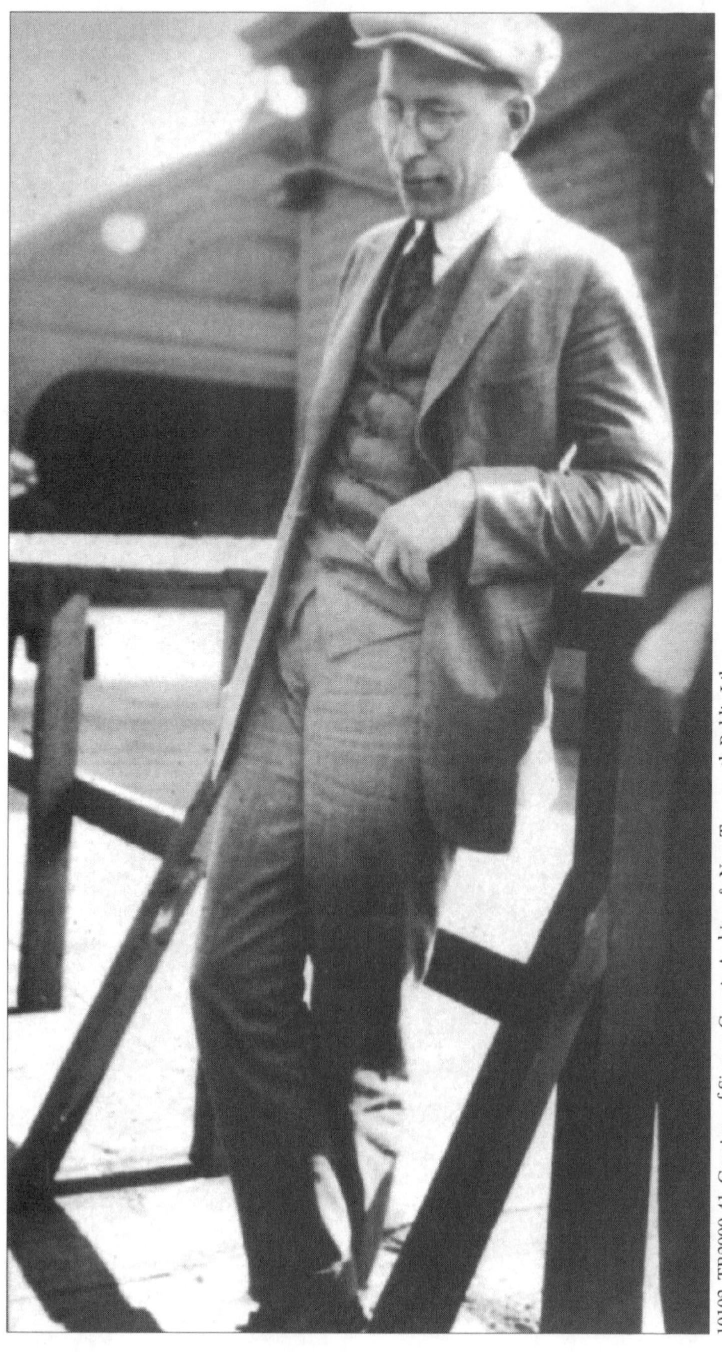

10102. TR2000-41. Courtesy of Simcoe County Archives & New Tecumseth Public Library.

A pensive, youthful Banting. In a few years
he will make a discovery that will change medicine forever.

1

A Brilliant Idea in the Middle of the Night

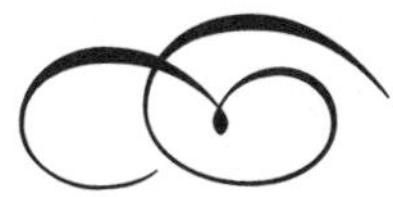

The doctor couldn't sleep. He was troubled. His medical practice in London, Ontario was going nowhere, and his girlfriend was thinking of leaving him.

It was just past midnight, on the last day of October, 1920. Because he had nothing better to do, he took out his paints and began painting a watercolour on a piece of cardboard.

The picture was of a house at night, in the snow. The house had one lighted window. He carefully painted shadows on the snow. The sound of the paint-brush was the only noise in the room.

He sat back and looked at the painting. It was a good painting. At least, he thought it was. He was pleased with the way the snow turned out. It wasn't easy to paint snow.

He began to sing an old war song called "Pack Up Your Troubles." He knew the words by heart. He sang under his breath, in a soft baritone. He liked the part about using a lucifer to light your fag. A lucifer was a sulphur match. He had troubles, all right. He stopped singing and lit a cigarette, a hand-rolled Piccadilly. He kept the cigarette between his lips while he painted.

The sign in front of the house where he lived at 442 Adelaide Street North said: Dr. F.G. BANTING. The front door had a shiny brass plate with his name on it. But the signs mocked him. In the last few months he had seen only a handful of patients.

He looked at his painting. It needed something else, maybe more snow. He painted some red into the window to make it look like the reflection from a fireplace.

He was engaged to Edith Roach, the daughter of a Methodist minister. She taught school a few miles away in the town of Ingersoll. It was embarrassing that she made more money than he did.

Like most women who worked, she planned to give up her job once she got married. She wanted to raise a family. No decent man in the 1920s would allow himself to be supported by his bride.

Edith wanted Fred to grow up, to settle down and earn a living. After all, he was twenty-eight. He wasn't young anymore. Whenever they saw each other they argued. Sometimes they were not sure they were still in love. Where was the man she once knew? He drank, smoked, and cursed. He didn't do that before the war.

It was bad enough that Banting had to pay for his house with money borrowed from his father, a hard-working farmer.

Banting had bought the house from a London shoe merchant, but the merchant still lived in the house with his wife. Banting agreed to let them stay while their new home was being built. The doctor had only two rooms: a bedroom and the front parlour. The parlour was also his office. The only furniture was a desk and wooden chair that he had borrowed from his father.

London was a community of sixty thousand people, about 150 kilometres west of Toronto. He had to remind himself that it was hard for a doctor to build up a practice in a new city. He had opened his office on July 1, four months ago. The patients were not exactly knocking down his door. To pass the time, he had started sketching and painting pictures.

His only patient in July was a man who wanted a prescription for alcohol so he could get drunk at a friend's wedding. Ontario was a "dry" province where drinking was prohibited. Banting wrote him the prescription. His fee was four dollars, his only income for the month.

To earn extra cash, Banting had taken a part-time job as a lecturer and demonstrator in surgery and anatomy at London's Western University. For this he received two dollars an hour.

Tonight he had to prepare for a talk he was giving his students. The subject was carbohydrate metabolism, the biochemical transformation of certain foods into energy for the body. He didn't know much about it. So he stubbed out his cigarette, put away his paints, cleaned his brushes, and reviewed what he planned to say.

He was aware that if you talked about carbohydrate metabolism, you also had to talk about a fatal disease called diabetes mellitus, "honey-sweet diabetes." As a physician, though, he wasn't particularly interested in diabetes and knew little about the subject. His knowledge came mainly from a lecture he had in medical school at the University of Toronto before he went off to war.

He tried to recall the details of his medical school lecture. He knew that food was digested by powerful enzymes from the pancreas, a jelly-like gland that was connected by ducts, or tubes, to the stomach. But the pancreas did something else, too. He remembered that a mysterious internal secretion within the pancreas supposedly regulated sugar in the bloodstream.

In the nineteenth century, German scientists discovered, by accident, that a dog became diabetic if its pancreas was removed. Excess sugar built up in the dog's urine, a condition called "glycosuria." The dog craved water and became listless, as if all the energy had drained from its body. Then the dog went into a coma and died.

Banting had seen diabetics before. The most severe form of diabetes, diabetes mellitus, struck children and young people. It was sometimes known as juvenile diabetes. The first symptoms were often an insatiable hunger and thirst. As the disease progressed, children lost almost all their body weight. Eating didn't help. They began to look like living skeletons. Death usually occurred within a year or two, but sometimes a child was gone in a week. There were one million people with diabetes in North America in 1920, and countless more around the world. The disease had never been conquered.

A condition that was probably diabetes mellitus appeared in the ancient writings of China and India. The description was the same one the Greeks and Romans reported – the patient urinates frequently, and the urine is sweet. The Greeks tested for diabetes by tasting the urine, or placing it next to an anthill to see if it attracted ants. The word "mellitus," honey-sweet, was coined to describe the disease.

Banting knew that "diabetes" came from the Greek word for "siphon." When people had diabetes, it was as if their lives were being siphoned away. The glucose from food was not absorbed into the cells and instead stayed in the blood. The sugar overload was so great, it spilled into the urine. That's why a diabetic's urine was sweet. The kidneys produced more urine than usual in an attempt to dilute the high levels of sugar. When the body lost this extra liquid, a terrible thirst was created. The craving for energy led to a hunger which no amount of eating could satisfy. Unable to obtain energy from food, the body tried to consume itself. Diabetic children were always so tired and hungry. They looked like victims of famine, and they were very quiet as death approached.

Life for diabetics was a constant struggle to ward off illness. Their skin became dry as paper. Their hair became brittle. They could go blind, or develop cataracts, a clouding of the lense of the eye. They tended to get lower-leg infections that formed gangrene, creating a horrible stench that permeated hospital wards. It often became necessary to amputate, but amputations were usually fatal because the wounds didn't heal. It was easy to see why diabetics were desperate for a cure. They grasped at anything. Hundreds of worthless patent medicines and fad diets, from potato cures to oatmeal cures, were on the market. But nothing could stop the disease.

Banting looked out the window at the deserted street. His reflection stared back at him. He was tall and big-boned, with a horsey face and wire-rimmed glasses. He had blue eyes and light-red hair. Edith said he had a good smile. But he wasn't smiling much these days.

He took a dog-eared anatomy book from the shelf. It was the same book he had in Europe when he was a medical officer in the Great War. He used to read it in the trenches while German shells whistled and exploded around him. Major L.C. Palmer, his superior officer, used to kid him about the way he studied. The other men had never seen anything like it. That Banting was something. He had guts. Not even the German guns could shake him. He was wounded in the right arm near Cambrai, France and received the Military Cross. That was two years ago. Now he was a doctor without any patients. A man who couldn't hold on to his girlfriend, a man with no future.

He opened the book. On the flyleaf was a date and the word "Cambrai." For a moment, he thought about the war. His Methodist parents brought him up to have a relationship with God, but the brutality of the conflict destroyed almost everything he had believed in. He didn't go to church anymore. Life in Canada had changed. There were more cars. Food was expensive. Women wanted to vote and have the same rights that men had.

He put the book back on the shelf and looked out the window. He remembered the farm where he grew up, near Alliston, Ontario. He loved the farm. He thought again about his lecture. Pancreas. What a strange word. His family used to eat animal pancreases. They were called sweetbreads and were fried or mixed into poultry stuffing.

In medical school, Banting was taught about the "undernutrition" therapy of Dr. Frederick Allen, an American who kept diabetic patients in a state of starvation as a way of holding down their blood sugar. Allen was lengthening their lives a little by reducing the impact of the disease. However, the patients eventually starved to death or succumbed to diabetes.

Allen did not believe that a pancreatic extract would ever be able to regulate blood sugar in a diabetic. No one did. It had been tried, and it didn't work. But that didn't bother Banting. He was blissfully ignorant. He didn't know anything about the background of Allen's method, or about diabetes research.

All Banting could think about were his problems with Edith and his lousy medical practice. He wished he could sleep. He began reading an article in a November 1920 medical journal he had just received in the mail, *Surgery, Gynecology and Obstetrics*.

The article was called, "The Relation of the Islets of Langerhans to Diabetes with Special Reference to

Cases of Pancreatic Lithiasis," by Dr. Moses Barron, an American pathologist who had become interested in the pancreas, and its relation to diabetes, while performing autopsies.

The Islets of Langerhans were a cluster of cells that floated within the pancreas like little islands. Scientists thought the islets had something to do with controlling blood sugar. Barron's article fascinated Banting. During the routine autopsy of a diabetic, Barron discovered that a pancreatic stone (lithiasis) had obstructed the main pancreatic duct to the stomach. What is more, he saw that the cells of the patient's pancreas had atrophied, or wasted away, while most of the cells in the Islets of Langerhans, within the pancreas, had remained healthy and intact.

Banting finished the article and dropped the medical journal to the floor. He took off his glasses. No matter how hard he tried, he couldn't get to sleep. He thought about the article, and the lecture he had to give, and rubbed his eyes. He put his face in his hands and cursed. The mantel clock ticked on.

At around 2:00 a.m., Banting sat straight up in his chair. He scribbled twenty-five words in his notebook: "Diabetus. Ligate pancreatic ducts of dog. Keep dogs alive till acini degenerate leaving Islets. Try to isolate the internal secretion of these to relieve glycosurea."

He misspelled diabetes and glycosuria. The spelling didn't matter. He'd always had trouble spelling. The important thing was the idea. Tie off the ducts that connect the pancreas to the stomach. Keep the dog alive until acini (pancreatic cells) degenerate, leaving behind the all-important Islets of Langerhans.

Try to isolate the internal secretion of these cells. Perhaps it could be used to relieve glycosuria, glucose in the urine, and the symptoms of diabetes.

Banting stayed up most of the night wondering if this mysterious secretion could be turned into an extract. If only it could be used to save diabetics.

In the morning he looked over his note. Maybe the idea was worth pursuing. He decided to try out his experiment. But the animal quarters at Western's medical building weren't big enough. Besides, there was a diabetes expert who was nearby, at the University of Toronto. His name was Professor J.J.R. Macleod, a Scotsman and respected researcher in the field of carbohydrate metabolism.

A week later, in November, while Banting was in Toronto for a wedding, he went to see Macleod. It was good to be back on the campus. He had gone to medical school here. But he had also failed his first year of university. He couldn't forget that.

Banting found Macleod's office and knocked on the door. "Enter, if you please," Macleod said in a thick Scottish accent.

The professor looked up from his desk and noticed Banting's scuffed shoes and threadbare jacket.

"How may I help you?"

"I am a physician and I have a research idea," Banting said.

"And what is your idea, Doctor..."

"Banting. Doctor Banting."

When Banting had finished describing his project, the professor said: "What is your research experience?"

"None, to speak of."

"Your published articles?"

"None."

"Other than this one article in the gynecology journal, your reading in the extensive diabetes literature of the past thirty years?"

"I'm afraid the answer is none."

Macleod sighed, looked down, and began reading from his pile of papers and correspondence.

Banting's face flushed with anger.

"Dammit," he said. "All I want are a few dogs for research. Maybe my idea is cockeyed. Maybe it's not. I'd like to find out."

Macleod stared at Banting. He didn't like the way this unruly Canadian talked, and he didn't expect him to succeed. For one thing, Macleod did not believe that an internal secretion of the pancreas could ever be isolated. In 1913, he had published a book on diabetes stating that very fact. Yet, he was intrigued by the idea that Banting wanted to work with atrophied or degenerated pancreases. No one had ever tried to develop an extract from a fully atrophied pancreas. The way Macleod saw it, Banting might as well follow the trail he was on, and besides, a failure in the laboratory might prove useful to diabetes researchers because it could eliminate one more step in the fruitless search for a treatment. He told Banting to wait and try the experiment the next summer.

A defeated Banting took the train home. He wondered if he should give up his medical practice, small as it was, and his part-time teaching job, for a questionable research project. When he mentioned the project to Edith, she told him to grow up and pay attention to his practice. He forgot about diabetes, and continued working in London as a physician.

ꝏ

The next spring, in March of 1921, Banting contacted Macleod to see if he remembered their interview. He did, and invited Banting to Toronto. Still, Banting wasn't sure. How was he supposed to earn a living? What if his idea was wrong? So far, his research was just words scribbled on a piece of paper.

For a while, he dropped diabetes altogether. He applied for a job as a medical officer to accompany an expedition to the Mackenzie River Valley in the Canadian North. But the job fell through at the last minute. If he had gone on the expedition, things might have been different. He might have returned to London, married Edith, and become a small-town medical practitioner.

He decided to plow ahead with the experiment, but only for the summer. On May 14, 1921, he took the train to Toronto. He rented a room in a Grenville Street boarding house that looked as if it had come from the island of Lilliput in *Gulliver's Travels*. He hung his sketches and watercolours on the walls. He paid two dollars a week for the 2.1 metre by 2.7 metre space.

Macleod provided him with ten dogs and a small laboratory on the top floor of the university's Medical

Building. He loaned him one of his student research assistants, Charley Best, a twenty-one-year-old graduate in physiology and biochemistry. He and another student, Clark Noble, had tossed a coin for the job, and Best won.

Best had grown up in Maine where his father, a Canadian from Nova Scotia, was a doctor. Best would help Banting with the research and perform blood and urine tests on the animals.

Banting and Best could not believe their eyes when they saw the lab. It looked as if it hadn't been used, or cleaned, in years. They washed the walls and ceiling, and scrubbed the wooden floor on their hands and knees.

On May 17, 1921, the two men, with Macleod, began their work on Banting's idea. The lab was next to the animal quarters and echoed with the sound of barking dogs.

The first dog was a brown spaniel. Macleod showed Banting how to operate on the dog and ligate, or tie off, the pancreas.

Macleod's office was in the same building, and he was consulted from time to time on the work. He gave Banting and Best instructions to keep careful records of their experiments before he left Toronto on June 14 for a three-month visit to his native Scotland. By the time the boat had sailed, the research was well underway.

When Banting and Best tried to operate on the dogs without Macleod, they ran into trouble. Some of the animals bled to death. Others died from infection. In two weeks, they had lost seven of the original ten dogs. After two months, seventeen dogs had died.

The work was slow. First, the dog had to be anesthetized and strapped to the operating table. Then Banting had to cut open the animal, carefully ligate the pancreatic ducts, and close the incision. Over several weeks, while the dog recovered, the pancreas would degenerate.

Banting believed it was important for the pancreas to degenerate. He did not want the external secretion of the pancreas, containing powerful ferments that digested food in the stomach, to destroy the "internal secretion" that went into the bloodstream to regulate blood sugar. It was this supposed internal secretion he was after.

On the face of it, the plan seemed simple. After several weeks, Banting would anesthetize the dog again and remove the degenerated pancreas. The gland would be chopped up and put into a laboratory mortar containing ice-cold Ringer's solution, a mixture of water and salts that was used in labs to preserve tissues. The pieces would then be ground up, and the solution filtered through cheesecloth to produce the extract. Warmed to body temperature, the extract would then be injected into diabetic dogs. These were dogs that had had their pancreases removed. This was the key to the experiment. Would the extract save their lives, and eventually the lives of diabetic humans?

In the 1920s, it was normal research practice to use animals in experiments. Banting loved animals, especially the dogs and horses on the farm. He saw animals as having been put on earth for the use of people. Now, as a doctor, he looked on them as special patients who would sacrifice their lives for others.

For centuries, diabetes had defeated the brightest scientists. The odds were stacked against Banting and Best. The research they were doing was held in such low regard, they were not even being paid.

2

Discovering Insulin

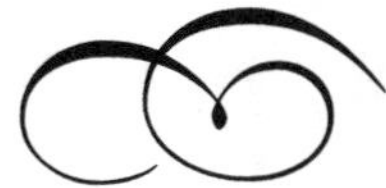

Toronto in the summer is hot and humid. The summer of 1921 was no different. The sun blazed down on the tar-and-gravel roof of the Medical Building where Banting and Best worked. To stay cool, Banting cut the sleeves off his lab coat.

Operating on the dogs wasn't easy. The pancreatic ducts were small and hard to find. The first dog they worked on died from an overdose of anesthetic. Banting had to be careful not to cut into major blood vessels. He often found himself drenched in blood.

Best, meanwhile, was using various chemical procedures to carefully measure the amount of sugar in the blood and urine of the animals.

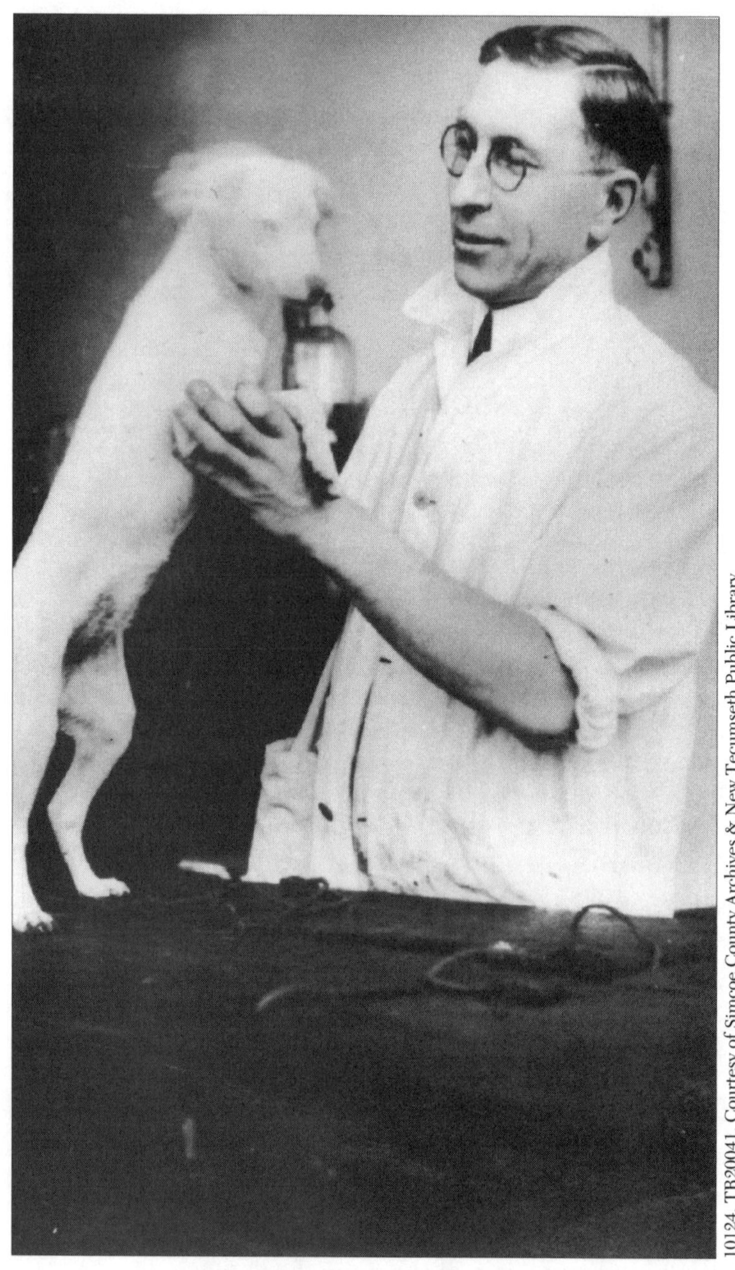

10124. TR20041. Courtesy of Simcoe County Archives & New Tecumseth Public Library.

Banting and one of his research dogs,
whom he thought of as special patients.

In the third week of June, with Macleod in Scotland, Banting had to work by himself. Best had gone to Ontario's Niagara region for ten days of militia training.

Like Banting, he was a war veteran. He had reached England as a sergeant when the war ended. He had graduated from the University of Toronto in physiology and biochemistry and was planning to study for his MA the next year. He and Banting had yet to produce any results, but he liked his summer job. Besides, four years ago, in 1917, one of his aunts had died from diabetes.

Banting found it frustrating to operate on the dogs and do the chemistry work while Best was away. He lost another dog during an operation to ligate its pancreas. It bled to death and he had to go out in the street and buy another hound. When he tried measuring for sugar in the dog's urine, he held the beaker up to the light and noticed that it was dirty. So was the rest of the glassware. He had a friend in the biochemistry building perform urine tests on another dog. The figures did not match up with the measurements Best had been getting. The dirty glassware had altered the results. Banting crossed out the rows of figures and numbers in his notebook and knew he'd have to talk to Best. If he didn't fix the problem, the research would fail.

After ten days, Best returned to the laboratory. The warm evening smelled of flowers and mowed lawns.

"Hullo, Dr. Banting! I had a splendid time."

Banting didn't respond.

"What's wrong? Is it the dogs?"

"I'll tell you what's wrong," Banting said. "Look at this."

He held out the notebook.

"The figures are all wrong. The experiments are ruined." He threw the notebook on the table. "Everything was dirty."

"What are you talking about? I washed the glassware," Best said.

"Not good enough. I told you if you wanted to work with me you'd have to show some interest but your work so far has been unsatisfactory. Maybe someone else would do a better job."

"It's just the bloody glassware," Best said, his voice trembling. "Why didn't you clean it when I was gone?"

"You can go to hell. I'll find someone else."

"You can't talk to me like that."

"Yes I can. Before you do another thing tonight you're going to throw away all the solutions that you've been using and wash every piece of glassware. Then I want you to make up new solutions. We have to provide consistent measurements for the samples we're taking or the research is useless. If the measurements are not accurate we won't be able to proceed. If the glassware is dirty, it will alter the results. Do you understand?"

Glaring into Banting's eyes, Best opened and closed his fist. Banting measured the height of Best's jaw. If there was going to be a fight, he wanted his first punch to be a good one. The two men stood there, sizing each other up. Finally, Best turned slowly and walked away.

He collected all the beakers, vials, and test tubes in the lab. He was angry, and threw them around in the sink. He washed and dried every single piece in the lab. Then he got to work. It was the first of many all-nighters for the student assistant. He'd soon learn that sleep was not important for Banting. After their encounter, they understood each other, and never argued like that again.

Best liked his summer research job. His girlfriend was living nearby, and when he wasn't working they'd play tennis or go swimming. Clark Noble, another of Macleod's students, was supposed to take over Best's job in July. Best wanted to stay. Noble agreed, and stepped out of the picture. He would always regret his decision.

Operating on the dogs was hard work. Sometimes the incisions did not heal, or the dogs that had their pancreases removed would not become diabetic because a tiny remnant of the gland would have been left inside the animal by mistake.

Banting and Best had to do everything. They even had to help the attendant clean out the dog cages. The stench in the laboratory was awful.

Time and time again they failed to come up with an extract that would lower a diabetic dog's blood sugar.

By July, Best was getting tired of the gruelling lab work. Banting cursed and swore in the stifling heat. The room stank and buzzed with flies. He wiped the sweat from his eyes so he could see to do the fine stitch-work that was required of delicate surgery.

But Banting refused to give up. When he ran out of dogs, he or Best would go out into the street and buy unwanted animals for around three dollars each. But they had to be careful. They didn't want the anti-vivisectionists to find out. These were well-intentioned people who opposed research experiments on dogs and other animals because they believed it was wrong for creatures to suffer pain and distress, whatever the reason.

While Toronto slept, the lights burned on in the Medical Building. Banting and Best laboured round the clock to find an extract that would keep diabetic dogs alive. They sang songs from the Great War to help themselves stay awake. They cooked their food over a Bunsen burner and sometimes, when they had to nap, curled up in the lab next to the barking animals.

One day in early August Banting and Best injected a diabetic collie with a new batch of extract and discovered that it actually drove down the dog's blood sugar. They called the extract, "isletin." They performed further experiments to confirm their findings.

On August 9, Banting wrote Macleod in Scotland, announcing that he and Best had an extract that reduced blood and urinary sugar and improved the clinical condition of diabetic dogs. Banting wondered if the extract would work on humans.

But there was one big problem. Producing "isletin" was slow, and it was difficult to make. Banting kept running out of extract.

Toward the end of August, Banting removed the pancreas from one of the dogs, a yellow collie known as

Number 92. When Number 92 became diabetic, they would try to keep her alive with extract. (The number referred to the university's record of dogs, not to the quantity or sequence of dogs used by Banting and Best.)

Banting didn't use gloves when he operated. He scrubbed with soap and water and used his bare hands. When the surgery was over, he looked at Number 92 as she lay sleeping on the recovery table. She reminded him of Collie, his boyhood pet.

The next day, when Banting returned to the lab, the dog was licking her incision to make it clean.

"Charley, she looks great," Banting said.

Th dog peered up at Banting, cocked her ears, and resumed cleaning her wound.

The operation was a success. It wasn't long before Number 92 developed diabetes mellitus. She was thirsty all the time, and kept urinating in her cage. They tested her urine for sugar. She became so listless she just lay on her side, breathing heavily. Banting looked at her eyes. They were cloudy and the corners were filled with pus. He snapped his fingers, but Number 92 didn't move. She was falling into a diabetic coma. Soon she would die.

"Charley, give me the isletin."

Banting drew about 2 cc of the extract into a syringe and injected the collie.

"That's a good girl," Banting said. He rubbed the site of the injection with his hand.

Best looked on.

"Dr. Banting, it's working. Look."

The effect was almost immediate. Slowly, she sat up on her haunches and shook her head, as if she had just awakened from a dream. Within a day, after several more injections, her eyes began to clear up, and the sugar in her urine disappeared. Banting and Best watched for symptoms that she was regressing, but she continued to improve. The injections were maintaining her health. The two men could hardly believe their eyes. The dog seemed to know what had happened. Whenever she saw Banting she'd stand up on her hind feet and place her paws in his hands and he would walk her around the lab, laughing.

Number 92 had no pancreas. According to every rule in the book, she should have been dead.

One day, about two weeks after the operation, when Banting asked Best for isletin, he heard the words: "There is no more." They had run out of extract.

Banting tried desperately to keep Number 92 alive. She began to exhibit all the symptoms of a diabetic. When she saw Banting she tried to walk to him, but staggered drunkenly, and collapsed to the floor. With tears in his eyes, Banting lifted her to the operating table. He spoke to her, and stroked her muzzle, and scratched behind her ears. But not even affection could rouse her.

On the hot, muggy night of August 31, she died as Banting looked helplessly on.

Banting had little money that summer. He had no salary and was paying the mortgage on an empty house in London. He couldn't borrow any more money from his parents. He earned a few dollars performing tonsillectomies and sold some of his medical instruments for spare cash. Once in a while he'd go to the Sunday night suppers put on by the Philathea Bible class of St. James Square Presbyterian Church. You could eat all you wanted, and it didn't cost a lot. Sometimes the girls from the Bible class would bring hot meals to the lab, or he'd fry eggs and heat up leftovers over a Bunsen burner.

When he did see Edith, they argued.

"Isn't time you settled down? You should hear what people back home are saying."

"I don't care what they say."

"You gave up your medical practice in London. You're acting like a boy."

Banting was stubborn. He refused to give up his research. He wondered why Edith couldn't see the importance of what he was doing. Finally, he decided to sell his house. He never wanted to see London again. He had his research idea there, but he had been lonely, and burdened with financial worries. Now he could devote himself to the job of finding a treatment for diabetes. He hoped Edith would understand, though he knew that neither she nor anyone else took the research as seriously as he did. By leaving London, he was, in a sense, preparing to leave Edith.

In September, Banting sold his house. He drove to London and picked up a few things in his car. It was a foggy morning. When he drove away he didn't look back.

On September 21, Macleod returned to Toronto from his vacation in Scotland. When Banting showed him the written results of the research for the past three months, Macleod was cautious. To Banting, it appeared that Macleod did not believe him.

"How do you know," the professor said, "that you have *actually* lowered the blood sugar in diabetic dogs?"

"It's right here," Banting replied. "We kept a record of everything."

"How do you know it wasn't something else?" Macleod inquired. "How do you know the isletin didn't merely dilute blood sugar levels in the animals? How do you know that when you removed the pancreas from a dog you didn't leave a little piece of the pancreas behind, a nodule, perhaps, that would somehow continue to do the work of the missing gland? Doctor Banting, you must be prepared to defend the results of your experiments."

Macleod told Banting to carry out further research to confirm his findings.

"You're crazy!" Banting exploded. "What are you talking about? Have you seen the conditions we work under? Have you forgotten we're not getting paid! I refuse to do any more work unless the conditions improve. I gave up everything in the world I had to do this research. I can go anywhere I want with my idea, and you know it! I'll go to New York!"

"Go ahead, Doctor."

"The damned lab floor is made of wood, and it's filthy. The place reeks of dog shit, and who cleans the cages? Me and Best, that's who."

Macleod didn't like Banting. He especially didn't like his unpredictable temper. The way Macleod saw it, Banting always showed up like bad weather.

"As I said, you're free to leave."

"For God's sake, Macleod!" Banting erupted. He stormed out of Macleod's office. When he saw Best, he complained bitterly.

"I can't believe he had the gall to question our findings," Banting said. "He wasn't even here! He was in Scotland! Hiking on the moors! We were doing all the work."

"Calm down, Dr. Banting. Don't fight with someone as powerful as Macleod. Remember, he's directing the research."

"I suppose he is." But Banting still wanted to sock Macleod in the jaw.

However, a few days later Macleod agreed to make some improvements to their working environment. Banting and Best were given a part-time lab boy to clean the dog cages and do the washing up. The operating room floor was tarred so it could be easily cleaned. In view of the results they had achieved, the university was persuaded to pay Banting and Best retroactively for their summer's research. Best got $170, the normal pay for a student assistant. Banting was paid $150 and, in order to continue working, was hired for the 1921-22 academic year as a special assistant in the pharmacology department at $250 a month. Banting and Macleod were on speaking terms again, for the time being, anyway.

By November, Banting realized that the method of making extract was taking far too long. Sometimes it took a month just to make a very small amount. Suddenly, he had an idea. Why not use fetal pancreases from a slaughterhouse? He remembered that farmers sometimes bred cattle before they were slaughtered. The farmers believed that pregnant cattle fetched a better price because they ate more and grew fatter. Banting knew that the islet cells of a pancreas developed early in fetal animals, and that these cells were supposed to produce an internal secretion that regulated blood sugar. He believed the digestive enzymes of the pancreas could not destroy this internal secretion, because the enzymes didn't function in fetal animals. The enzymes weren't needed to digest food until after birth. He concluded that it would be easier to produce the extract he needed from the pancreas of a fetal calf.

He and Best drove to the William Davies Company's slaughterhouse in northwest Toronto and cut out the pancreases from nine calf fetuses. They took the fetal glands back to the lab and used them to produce an extract that was successful at reducing the blood and urinary sugar of diabetic dogs. Now they wouldn't have to go through the complicated, time-consuming procedure of operating on dogs, ligating their pancreases, and waiting for the glands to degenerate. All the fetal pancreas they needed could be obtained from slaughterhouses. Now they would have plenty of extract. For Banting and Best, it was the beginning of a new stage in their work.

Word of the research began to spread. Dr. Elliott Joslin, a prominent diabetologist in Boston, heard about their findings. He was using the "undernutrition" or "starvation" method of Dr. Frederick Allen, the accepted method for treating diabetes in 1921. Allen ran the Physiatric Institute, a diabetic clinic in Morristown, New Jersey.

Under Allen's method, severe diabetics went on a liquid fast until their blood sugar was lowered. Their diet was gradually built up to a minimal level, with strict measuring of all foods. When sugar appeared in the urine, the food limit was reached. The patients were forced to stay on a "starvation" diet consisting of foods such as crusts and boiled fruit. There was always a strong temptation to break the diet. Even diabetics who followed the diet eventually died, starving to death or succumbing to the disease. The good thing about the method was that it gave diabetics a little more time to stay alive. There was always the faint hope that a treatment for diabetes would be found, but no one knew when that would be.

Joslin was a great physician who had seen too many diabetics die. He hoped that a treatment had been discovered in Toronto. It was awful to have to stand by helplessly and watch as children slipped into a coma. The breathing of the patient was loud and deep, a phenomenon that physicians called "air hunger." The pulse was small. The breath had a strong fruit-like odour, which was the smell of "ketones," resulting from the breakdown of stored fat in the body. Death occurred within hours. There was nothing the parents or the physician could do.

Joslin wrote Macleod to inquire about the research. In November, Macleod replied that the work at the University of Toronto might be of real value in the treatment of diabetes and that they were hurrying along the experiments as fast as possible.

In November, Banting injected himself subcutaneously (under the skin) with the extract. He had no reaction, demonstrating, at least, that the extract was not toxic to healthy humans.

Macleod showed Banting and Best how to mix a pancreas with alcohol, evaporate the mixture, and redissolve the residue in a salt solution, producing an injectable extract.

Banting eventually discovered he was able to produce an extract with whole beef pancreas, which meant that he and Best did not have to rely on calf fetuses. As long as there was access to a slaughterhouse, there would always be a source for the extract.

At Banting's suggestion, Macleod invited J.B. (Bert) Collip to join the group working on the extract. Collip was from Belleville, Ontario, the son of a florist. He was the same age as Banting. He started working with Banting and Best in December, 1921. Collip was an inventive biochemist whose lab was in a building that was several blocks away. The four men were now working as a team, meeting for lunch and planning experiments.

On December 22, Collip made a momentous discovery. He knew that when a person has diabetes, the liver's ability to store glucose in the form of glycogen is impaired. The storing of glycogen is one of the body's most important functions. Glycogen is stored energy, and the liver will turn it into sugar and release it into the bloodstream if a person has a need for some of this energy. Collip tested to see if the extract could restore this lost function in a diabetic rabbit. It did. But would it work on people?

Banting contacted Joe Gilchrist, a former medical school classmate who had diabetes, and whose health was rapidly declining. In December, Gilchrist swallowed some "isletin," but it had no effect. The extract did not work when taken orally. To save lives, it would have to be injected.

On December 30, Banting presented the results of the last few months' work to the American Physiological Society conference at Yale University. His paper was called, "The Beneficial Influences of Certain Pancreatic Extracts on Pancreatic Diabetes."All the important American doctors and researchers in diabetes were there. Banting became almost mute with fear. He had never spoken to such an important group before. He spoke haltingly. Macleod had to step in during the question period and defend the research.

On the train back to Toronto, Banting stayed up all night and brooded. He had worked month after month under the most gruelling conditions, but it seemed as if Macleod was getting the credit. He decided that Macleod was trying to steal his work, and he began to suspect Collip, too, because Collip and Macleod were friends.

Less than two weeks later, on January 11, 1922, Banting and Best took their extract across College Street to Toronto General Hospital. They did not have clinical privileges at the hospital, so they waited outside the ward while a house physician injected 15 cc of the mud-coloured "isletin" extract into a fourteen-year-old charity patient named Leonard Thompson, 7.5 cc into each buttock. The boy's diabetes and "undernutrition" diet had reduced him to thirty kilograms. When he breathed, the odour of diabetic acidosis, a smell like rotten fuit, filled the room. Thompson's blood sugar dropped temporarily, but the extract produced no clinical benefit. A sterile abscess, caused by the impurities in the extract, developed at the site of one of the injections. He was the first human diabetic to be injected with the extract.

Under Macleod's direction, Collip tried to improve the extract by purifying it further. He mixed whole beef pancreas with alcohol, mixing countless batches, using endless combinations. This was hit-and-miss research, but Collip was a chemistry artist, a genius in the lab. He realized, sometime in January, that the extract sometimes caused convulsions in rabbits because it reduced blood sugar too far, causing a hypoglycemic reaction now known as "insulin shock." (The antidote for the reaction is to give the patient sugar.)

On January 16, 1922, Collip succeeded in finally purifying the extract. He did this by gradually increasing the concentration of alcohol in the mixtures. The active principle in the extract stayed in the solution at higher and higher concentrations of alcohol, while the remaining substances in the extract precipitated out or were extracted by centrifuging. At a certain concentration of alcohol, the active principle itself was precipitated out – this was insulin.

On January 23, Leonard Thompson, slipping into a coma, was given 5 cc of the purified extract. He revived almost immediately. A few hours later he was given two injections of 10 cc each. His glycosuria almost disappeared. His ketonuria, ketones in the urine, vanished. (Ketones are produced when the body breaks down its own fat supply to use as energy when it is unable to use sugar. Ketones give off a strong, fruity smell. A buildup of ketones is harmful to the body.) The extract had been purified by Collip but was the result of the work of all four men, based on Banting's idea.

But no one was celebrating. The relations among the men soured. One evening, toward the end of January, Banting saw Collip in the Medical Building.

"Whoa there," he said. "What's the hurry?"

"I'm late," Collip said, smiling.

"You've been busy," Banting said. "That was tremendous, purifying the extract. The Thompson boy, it was all just tremendous."

"Thanks, Fred. Have to run."

"One more thing," he said. "How did you do it? How did you purify the extract?"

"Can't tell you that."

"Can't tell? What do you mean can't tell?"

Collip explained that he had told Macleod, and that the secret was safe with him. Macleod, he said, had agreed he did not have to disclose his method.

Moreover, Banting thought he heard him say that he wanted to take out a patent on the process. That was too much for Banting. He went wild with rage. He grabbed Collip by the lapels of his overcoat, lifted him, and threw him in a chair. The men struggled. Collip tried to protect his face with his arms. He couldn't escape. Banting was too strong.

Best grabbed Banting and with great effort pulled him away. He was afraid that Collip would be seriously injured.

After this incident, Macleod made everyone sign a peace agreement. Banting, Best, and Collip agreed to work under Macleod's general direction and cooperate with the university's new Connaught Antitoxin Laboratories to develop the potent extract. They promised not to have the extract individually patented.

Meanwhile, the name "isletin" was changed to "insulin." Banting agreed with Macleod that "isletin" was hard to pronounce and didn't have as much significance as "insulin," which comes from "insula," a Latin root word that means "island." It refers to the islets (little islands) of Langerhans, the cells in the pancreas which produce the secretion that regulates blood sugar.

The word "insulin" was first publicly used in a paper Macleod presented to the Association of American Physicians in Washington, D.C., on May 3, 1922. He summarized the work and went over the results. Dr. Joslin and Dr. Allen, the famed American diabetologists, sat awestruck in the audience.

Macleod told the physicians it had been demonstrated conclusively in Toronto that a pancreatic extract known as "insulin" could control the metabolism of diabetic animals and diabetic humans. For the first time in history, there was a substance that could be used in the treatment and control of diabetes. Macleod warned, though, that producing insulin on a large scale could prove difficult.

The audience of doctors, the best practitioners in North America, realized they were listening to one of the greatest achievements in modern medicine. As a group, they stood at the end of Macleod's address to honour the discovery.

Insulin would change medicine forever. Banting and Best, under Macleod's direction, had begun their work in a dingy lab only a year before, on May 17, 1921. No one had expected them to succeed. Collip eventually became part of the team.

The names of the researchers were listed alphabetically in Macleod's paper. Banting's name came first, then Best. But they were not at the meeting. They were back in Toronto. They said they couldn't afford the trip. But Banting probably just didn't want to go. He was still mad at Collip and Macleod, and besides, he didn't care about applause. He had always wanted to heal broken lives, ever since he was a boy on the farm, and now he was living his dream.

When Macleod was in Washington for the announcement, Banting was in his boarding house room drinking lab alcohol diluted with water. The alcohol was the same stuff that was used to make the extract. He drank because he was lonely, and to help him fall asleep. The other boarders could hear him singing "It's A Long, Long Way To Tipperary" and other songs that were popular in the Great War. After a few drinks, he began to talk to himself. He talked about Edith, whom he could never please, and the war, and insulin. He smoked his pipe, and read Sherlock Holmes. As far as he was concerned, insulin was his idea. It was a brilliant idea. He was in charge, and the others had come along for the ride to give him directions in case he got lost.

He had broken up with Edith two months ago. Now perhaps he'd have more time to visit his parents. The farm where he grew up, and where his parents still lived, was near Alliston, about sixty kilometres north of Toronto. There, on the farm, time stood still. His father, William, still ploughed the land and harvested crops and sawed trees that had been felled by lightning. Banting's mother, Margaret, still washed and cooked, and churned the butter. They knew Fred was a good boy.

3

The Luckiest Boy in the World

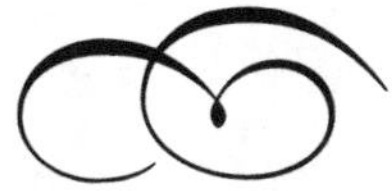

Frederick Grant Banting was born on November 14, 1891, in the downstairs bedroom of his family's farmhouse. He had a sister and three brothers. A fourth brother, a baby, died of whooping cough in 1886.

Fred was the youngest in the family – four years younger than his sister, seven years younger than his next oldest brother. His playmates on the forty-hectare farm were the dogs and other farm animals.

His mother tucked him in bed at night with the prayer: "Now I lay me down to sleep, and pray the Lord my soul to keep."

There was a big clock on a shelf above the kitchen table. The glass door of the clock was painted with

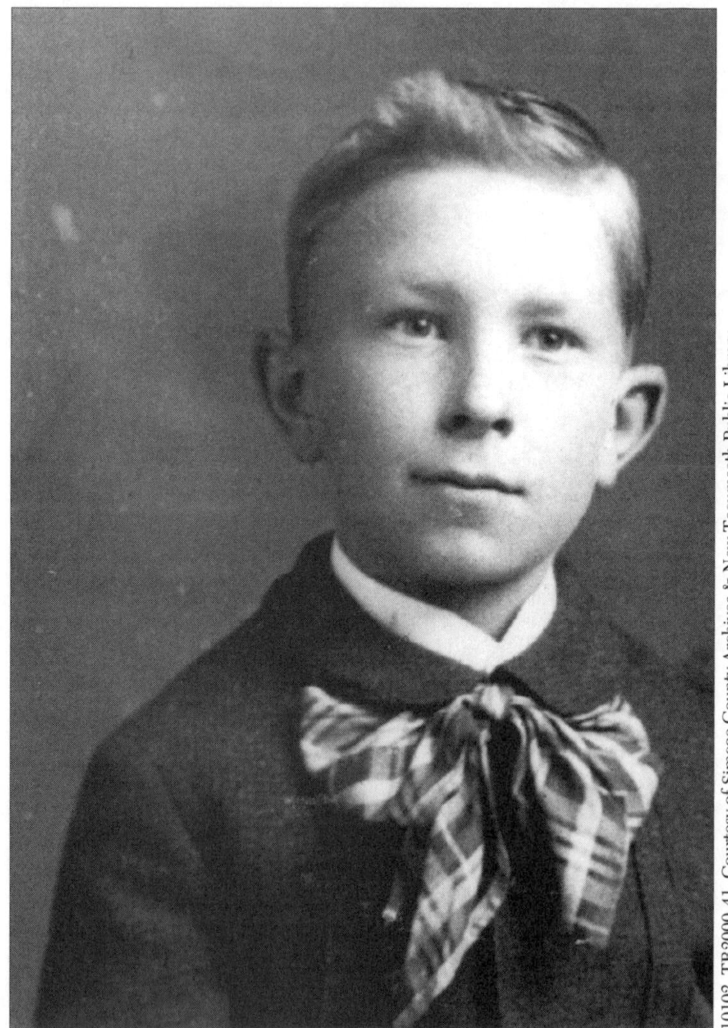

10102. TR2000-41. Courtesy of Simcoe County Archives & New Tecumseth Public Library.

Young Banting when he was living on the farm in Ontario. In only a few more years, he would decide he wanted to become a doctor.

palm trees and a faded moon. Fred's mother kept a little bottle of rat poison behind the clock door. He loved to stare at that moon, and those trees. To Fred, the clock moon was as real as the moon that floated above the fields of Alliston.

The Bantings were God-fearing Methodists of British descent. They prayed every day. They believed in the value of honesty and hard work. In the morning, after breakfast, Fred's father, a tall, bearded man, read from the Bible. Afterwards, the entire family knelt on the kitchen floor and recited the Lord's Prayer. On Sunday mornings the family went to church. In the afternoon Fred attended Sunday School, where his father taught one of the classes.

Fred was shy. Every day he walked about four kilometres to school. It was a long, lonely trek from his parents' farm to the school, in the village of Alliston, across the Boyne River and the rolling countryside.

The farm was heaven to the boy. In the winter he skated on the Boyne and went maple sugaring. In the summer he went fishing and ran barefoot through the fields with the family dog, Collie, who only went into the farmhouse when it thundered, to hide under a dark stairwell until the storm had passed. The doghouse, under a cherry tree in the backyard, was lined with a buffalo robe in winter, and it had a little porch to keep the snow from blowing in.

At ploughing time the boy rode on the broad back of the Clydesdale that worked the land. Afterwards he helped his father remove the heavy harness that smelled of leather and horse sweat.

The farmhouse was built on the crest of a hill. From the top of the hill, Fred could see the houses of Alliston, and the trees which lined the banks of the Boyne. To the west were the Blue Mountains. To the east, about twenty-five kilometres away, was Lake Simcoe.

If the farm was paradise, then school was hell. Fred hated school. He ate his lunch in the hallway at school or by the old fairgrounds in town. The other children went home at noon for lunch. But not Fred. The farm was too far away. When he ate at the fairgrounds he was sometimes so lonely he cried.

He lived in terror of being asked a question in class. Even if he knew the answer, he couldn't seem to get it out. He couldn't spell, either. No matter how hard he tried, he made mistakes. He filled notebooks with spelling exercises, sometimes writing a word a hundred times, but it didn't help. When he had to spell a word, he guessed. It was a problem he'd have all his life.

The Bantings were proud of their farm. Fred's mother kept the house spotless. In winter, fat scrapings were saved from beef and pork. The fat was mixed in the spring with lye and fireplace ash and other ingredients, and boiled down to make soap. The soap was used to clean the wooden chairs and tables and floors and even the doorstep of the house. Fred liked to watch his mother make soap. He was fascinated with the mixing, boiling, and stirring that went into soap production.

The centre of the family library was a well-thumbed Bible. There was also a copy of *The Pilgrim's*

Progress, John Bunyan's seventeenth-century classic about the adventures of Christian and his battles with evil, temptation, and despair. Fred loved that book. He loved the pictures of the giants, dragons, and monsters the hero encounters on the way to the Celestial City. Like *Gulliver's Travels* and *Robinson Crusoe*, Bunyan's book was written for adults but was also popular with children, who especially liked the illustrated editions.

The Banting library also contained novels by Sir Walter Scott and Charles Dickens, and poetry by William Wordsworth. One of the books had a long title: *The Bible Looking-Glass, Reflector, Companion and Guide to the Great Truths of the Sacred Scriptures, and Illustrating the Diversities of Human Character and the Qualities of the Human Heart, Profusely Illustrated by Object Teaching Pictures, Showing the Pain and Misery Resulting from Vice and the Peace and Happiness Arising from Virtue*.

In the evening, the family gathered round the kitchen stove and listened as Fred's father read aloud from one of the novels.

Above the kitchen was the room where the family bathed. A hole had been cut in the floor to let in heat from the kitchen stove below. Fred lay on the floor and peeked through the hole to watch his father or just listen to the words from the book while imagining that he was in the world created by the novelist.

On this particular evening, the wind was blowing so hard the house shook. But Fred didn't mind. In the dull, red glow of the stove fire, his father opened *The Old Curiosity Shop*, by Charles Dickens, and began where he had left off the night before, in chapter seventy:

As it grew dusk, the wind fell; its distant moanings were more low and mournful; and as it came creeping up the road, and rattling covertly among the dry brambles on either hand, it seemed like some great phantom for whom the way was narrow, whose garments rustled as it stalked along. By degrees it lulled and died away; and then it came on to snow.

The flakes fell fast and thick, soon covering the gound some inches deep, and spreading abroad a solemn stillness. The rolling wheels were noiseless; and the sharp ring and clatter of the horses' hoofs, became a dull, muffled tramp. The life of their progress seemed to be slowly hushed, and something death-like to usurp its place…

His father read on. Fred lay upstairs, lulled nearly to sleep by the heat of the stove and the sound of his father's words.

Before he knew it, his father had begun the next chapter, where the old man cannot distinguish spirits from people, and refuses to believe that Nell, his granddaughter, is dead.

The old man turned slowly towards him: and muttered, in a hollow voice, "This is another! – how many of these spirits there have been tonight!"

"No spirit, master. No one but your old servant. You know me now, I am sure? Miss Nell – where is she – where is she?"

"They all say that!" cried the old man. "They all ask the same question. A spirit!"

"Where is she?" demanded Kit. "Oh tell me but that – but that, dear master!"

"She is asleep – yonder – in there."

"Thank God!"

"Ay! Thank God!" returned the old man. "I have prayed to Him many, and many, and many a livelong night, when she has been asleep. He knows. Hark? Did she call?"

"I heard no voice..."

The elder Banting stopped. Overcome with emotion, he couldn't go on. He lay the book on his knees, drew a handkerchief from his pocket, and wiped his eyes. He handed the book to his wife, who continued without a pause, until she had finished the chapter:

"... It is not on earth that Heaven's justice ends. Think what it is, compared with the World to which her young spirit has winged its early flight, and say, if one deliberate wish expressed in solemn terms above this bed could call her back to life, which of us would utter it!"

After each reading, the family would talk about the characters in the novel as if they were real people.

Tonight Fred wanted an encore. He shouted through the hole: "Father, read some more!"

"More is it you want? Or do you want to delay your bedtime?"

His sister and brothers laughed.

"I want to hear about Quilp!" Fred shouted.

Quilp was the evil dwarf in the book who ate hard-boiled eggs, shells and all, and gigantic prawns with the heads and tails still on.

"Fred doesn't want to go bed because he's afraid of the bears!" one of the brothers shouted.

"The bears under his bed!"

"There ain't no bears!" Fred yelled.

"How do you know?" his father asked.

"I seen there ain't no bears."

The entire family laughed.

"All right, I'll read," his father said. "It's Quilp, then off to bed with you."

It was the chapter where Quilp's mother-in-law, under the impression that he has drowned, dictates a description of the corpse to Sampson Brass, his attorney. The dwarf tries to overhear the conversation.

"Respecting his legs now –"

"Crooked, certainly," said Mrs. Jiniwin.

"Legs crooked," said Brass, writing as he spoke. "Large head, short body, legs crooked –"

"Very crooked," suggested Mrs. Jiniwin...

"A question now arises in relation to his nose."

"Flat," said Mrs. Jiniwin.

"Aquiline!" cried Quilp, thrusting in his head, and striking the feature with his fist. "Aquiline, you hag. Do you see it? Do you call this flat? Do you? Eh!"

Fred was satisfied. It was time for bed, and prayers.

In the fall of 1903, Fred was almost twelve. It was the beginning of a new school year.

The Banting family was in the kitchen. Fred's father had just led the family in the Lord's Prayer. Morning was the time for spiritual contemplation, and reading from the Bible or *The Pilgrim's Progress*.

The elder Banting took *The Pilgrim's Progress* from the shelf and began to read. Fred was fascinated by the adventures of Christian, the hero of the book. But he had something else on his mind right now. His mother had given him a new pair of boots. They were too big for his older sister Essie, but they fit Fred perfectly. He would have to wear them to school. High-button girl's boots!

His father opened the book to a section called, "The Valley of the Shadow of Death." He cleared his throat, and began:

Now, morning being come, he looked back, not out of desire to return, but to see, by the light of the day, what hazards he had gone through in the dark. So he saw more perfectly the ditch that was on the one hand, and the quag that was on the other; also how narrow the way was which led betwixt them both. Also now he saw the hobgoblins, and satyrs, and dragons of the pit, but all afar off; for after break of day they came not nigh, yet they were discovered to him, according to that which was written, "He discovereth deep things out of darkness, and bringeth to light the shadow of death."

Fred shuddered. He didn't know which was worse: having to wear girl's boots to school, or having to walk through the valley of death with its monsters, devils, and shadows.

On the way to school, he took the boots off and left them under the Scotch Line bridge over the Boyne. He went to school barefoot. Every day, on his way home, he put them back on again. He dragged them in the dirt. He kicked them against the rocks. He dunked them in the river. Nothing wore them down. They were indestructible. He was the only student who still went to school barefoot.

Finally, one day in October, it snowed. Now he had to wear the boots or his feet would freeze. In class, he kept his feet hidden under his desk. No one noticed. But he ran into "Smack," the school bully, a boy who smoked and stole candy from younger children.

"Hey, boys, Fred's got new boots."

"Never you mind," Fred said, walking away.

"Give us a look-see of them new girly boots."

"I'm tellin' you, Smack."

"Girly boots, girly – ."

The brawl was on. They punched, and rolled in the snow, and when it was over the bully had given up in tears. No one dared tease Fred now. He had won the right to wear the awful boots.

A few days later, when he was in town with his mother, he tried to hide behind her skirt so no one would notice the boots.

"Why are you behaving like that?"

"The boots, Mother."

"Do they hurt your feet?"

"They're girl's boots."

"Why didn't you say something before?"

"Didn't think to."

"Let's go in here and buy a pair of proper boots."

Most farm boys dropped out of school before taking the entrance examinations for high school. The boys who continued their education sometimes went on to the Ontario Agricultural College in Guelph. High school graduates from the country rarely went on to university.

One day, on the way home from school, Fred stopped to watch two men shingling a roof. Their scaffold broke, and the men fell to the ground. Fred ran for the doctor. While the doctor tended their cuts and broken bones, Fred watched in admiration. He decided then and there he wanted to be a doctor. Fred's parents wanted him to become a Methodist minister, but he believed the greatest service to others was found in the medical profession.

Banting was now a strapping nineteen-year-old. He was tall, and built like a rugby player. He enrolled in the general arts course at Victoria College of the University of Toronto, the largest university in Canada. Victoria College was a Methodist college, and Fred's Methodist minister from home went with him on the first day to register. Toronto was a big, sophisticated city with 500,000 people. It was not at all like Alliston or the surrounding townships.

Fred failed his first year at university. He passed Latin, English, Mathematics, Biology, and Greek-and-Roman history, but German and French were too much for him. He was not allowed to enter his second year until he passed his failed language courses.

He wanted to study medicine. He petitioned the university and was allowed to enter medical school on the condition that he make up his failed courses while pursuing his medical studies. He spent the spring and summer of 1912 helping his father on the farm.

Fred and Edith met in the summer of 1911, the year her family moved to Alliston. Her father was a Methodist minister. The young couple saw each other at church picnics, and went boating on the Boyne. In the winter they enjoyed skating and sleigh-riding. They didn't go dancing. Some Methodists frowned on dancing as sinful. But Fred didn't like to dance anyway. He was clumsy. He might as well have had two left feet.

In September, 1912, Fred left Alliston for Toronto and entered the first year of the University of Toronto's five-year course in medicine. Doctors in North America were respected. But it wasn't always like that. In the early part of the nineteenth century, medicine had a bad reputation. Doctors were often seen as butchers who inflicted pain on their victims. Sometimes doctors bled their patients to death, or poisoned them with bogus compounds laced with mercury or arsenic. By the early 1920s, most doctors were using vaccines and had adopted antiseptic procedures. Anesthesia had revolutionized surgery. But medicine still had a long way to go. One of the biggest killers, diabetes, had terrorized people for centuries. When Fred was in medical school, the accepted treatment for diabetics was to control their blood sugar by keeping them in a state of starvation. No matter how diabetes was treated, the patients always died. Diabetes was a death sentence.

The medical building at the University of Toronto was opened in 1903 by world-renowned Canadian physician and medical teacher, Sir William Osler. The university had one of the largest medical schools in North America.

Banting studied hard, but he was only an average medical student. To relax, he skated and played rugby and baseball. Edith's aunt and uncle lived in Toronto. She stayed with them while she took language courses at the university's Victoria College. She and Fred often studied together.

From time to time he took the train home for the weekend. His sister would meet him at the station and they'd walk over to the horses waiting in the church shed. He couldn't wait to see his favourite horse.

"Mollie?" he called.

Halfway down the row the horse turned her head and whinnied in response.

He greeted Mollie with a big hug around the neck. He talked to her, and she seemed to talk back in her own language as if she understood every word and nuance of emotion.

Life seemed idyllic, but the world was changing. The British Empire declared war on Germany in 1914. Fred wanted to fight. But he was rejected twice because of poor eyesight. He tried again and was accepted into the Canadian Army Medical Service. He spent the summer of 1915 in training camp in Niagara Falls before returning to Toronto to complete his fourth year in medicine. Doctors were needed for the war. To speed up the education of doctors, the university condensed the fifth year of Fred's class, offering a special summer session in 1916.

In March, 1917, Banting sailed from Halifax to England. In May, he was posted to a hotel on the

English seaside that had been turned into a hospital for soldiers who had been maimed or blinded by poison gas.

In June, 1918, he was transferred to a Canadian hospital in France to treat wounded men. Then he was sent to a Canadian field ambulance unit in the Amiens-Arras sector, where he cleaned and dressed wounds before the men were sent back to base hospitals.

Banting's division sometimes had to take over some of the abandoned German dugouts. These were large, reinforced trenches big enough to walk around in. The dugouts were turned into dressing stations and operating theatres to treat wounded soldiers. Any structure close to the front line – a dugout, a farmhouse, a barn – might be turned into a makeshift hospital.

The medical corps was constantly exposed to enemy gunfire. The men in the corps worked long hours without rest. They worked at night by the light of smoky lanterns. Battle casualties in the corps were high.

The shelling seemed to go on forever. Banting was exhausted. Finally, one night, there was relative calm. The firing of big guns was sporadic. Banting and Major L.C. Palmer, his superior officer, stood in one of the unprotected doorways of a captured German dugout. They had spent the day applying tourniquets, amputating limbs when necessary, and performing operations. Now and then a German flare lit up the sky. Banting puffed on his pipe. The scene was almost beautiful. Clouds of poison gas drifted across the horizon. The glow from distant fireworks filtered through the deadly fog like light through a prism, colouring the sky.

Suddenly, a big German shepherd appeared out of nowhere and headed straight for them. There were standing orders to kill or capture these runner dogs, which were used to carry messages.

"Look out," Palmer said.

"I see it," Banting whispered.

The dog stopped, looked at the men, and growled. Palmer reached for his pistol but the dog ran quickly past them into the candlelit dugout.

"Damn, she was fast," Banting said.

"Like a bloody ghost."

"Let's go get her."

The officers followed the animal down. She stood in a corner, panting. Palmer poured out some water from a canteen. Warily, the animal drank. The men saw that the shepherd wasn't carrying any messages. They returned to the top of the steps, and Banting relit his pipe. The dog quietly lay down between them. Suddenly, the animal howled and threw itself down the steps. They turned to look. Just then the battleworks was hit by a shell, and the men were thrown to the ground. They covered their heads to protect themselves from the rocks and mud that fell from the sky in the aftermath of the explosion. They looked at each other. Another close call.

"It was the dog," Palmer said.

"A damn lucky dog," Banting said.

"Lucky for us."

Next day the dog was taken away.

"That shepherd saved our lives," Banting said to the driver when the dog was loaded on to a truck. "Take care of her."

❧

In August, 1918, Banting was posted to the front lines as a medical officer to the 44th Battalion, 4th Canadian Division. As a battalion medical officer, he was the doctor for the men in the unit and was the first to treat the wounded in action.

In September, his unit joined the attack around Cambrai, in northern France. The desolate landscape was littered with dead soldiers in various positions of repose, as if they were sleeping, and the putrid remains of horses and mules. He was waiting to clear his wounded from one of the aid posts when the Germans counter attacked. A German soldier with a long-barreled pistol, the type that was issued to ground troops, burst through the doorway. A shot rang out, and the German dropped. Banting looked around. The shot was fired by a sergeant whose foot he had amputated. He was sitting up on a stretcher, holding a carbine. Banting knelt by the German, checked the wound, and felt for a pulse. Nothing. He turned to the sergeant.

"Thanks," he said.

"Don't mention it, Captain. I didn't want Jerry to take my other foot."

Banting moved his patients to another station. He barely had time to eat or sleep.

Before it was over, forty thousand men would die at Cambrai. It was a bloodbath, the first time in the history of warfare that tanks were used en masse.

Nearly five hundred British tanks led the advance along the front. Men, artillery, horses, and tanks concentrated around Bourlon Ridge to the west of

Cambrai. The big tanks got bogged down in the mud, suffered mechanical failure, or were smashed by German artillery at close range.

Day and night the fighting continued. It was up to the medical corpsmen to patch up the wounded, amputate limbs, or make a declaration of death so the soldier's loved ones could be notified back home.

Learning that a Canadian medical officer had been hit, Banting took a party of stretcher-bearers and made his way to the front to help with the wounded. He had to cross open terrain, where he was an easy target for German machine guns. When some of his men were wounded, he stopped to bandage them but was pinned down by the fire. Each time he tried to stand, the guns started blazing. He lay on his stomach and watched soldiers on horseback charge the Germans. With every cannon burst the earth vomited up mud and horses and soldiers. When the cavalry leader and his horse were knocked to the ground by an explosion, the horse got up and began to gallop away. But the horse stopped, returned to the officer, and allowed him to climb back on. As the horseman rode to safety, Banting marvelled at the animal's loyalty and affection. For a moment he remembered Mollie, his favourite horse, and how she used to greet him on weekends when he came home from medical school. Then a machine-gun burst brought him back to the war. He lay flat while bullets whizzed overhead and raked the ground around him.

In late September, 1918, the Allied forces pushed forward. Banting and Palmer were in charge of a dressing station that was housed in a partially demolished barn, in a place called Lilac Farm, near Cambrai. An artillery officer, without Palmer's permission, had set up a cannon in the barnyard and was firing at the Germans. The Germans were determined to put the gun out, and shells rained all around. The German prisoners in the farmhouse began to grow nervous. One of the shells landed in the barnyard and a piece of shrapnel decapitated a German prisoner. An L-shaped fragment from the same shell wounded Banting, severing an artery and lodging between the bones of his right forearm. Blood pumped from the wound. Palmer applied a tourniquet and quickly operated, removing the fragment.

He said: "There's an ambulance here to take you to the nearest clearing station."

"Like hell," Banting growled. "I'm not going. You don't have enough men as it is. Besides, it's just a scratch."

Palmer could see that Banting might go into shock. He had lost a lot of blood.

The order came to secure Cambrai, which had just been taken from the enemy. The major had to leave to set up a field hospital in the town.

He reminded Banting to get in the ambulance. But instead of doing as he was told, Banting stayed at Lilac Farm and treated the wounded.

When Palmer arrived in the town, the Germans counter-attacked. He was forced to hide in the cellar of a building. The battle seesawed. Finally the British drove the Germans out.

The next day, when Palmer returned to the farm, he found the wounded Banting still tending to patients.

"This time you're going," Palmer said. "Don't disobey my orders again."

Banting nodded. He was so exhausted he could barely stand. His arm was throbbing. He barely made it to the loaded ambulance. He climbed into the front seat beside the driver and fell asleep. The roads were rough from heavy shelling, and the ambulance bounced along. Banting winced in pain each time the vehicle hit a pothole. As the truck pulled up to the clearing station, the wound began to hemorrhage. Doctors stopped the bleeding and gave Banting a shot of morphine. In the last twenty-four hours he had hardly eaten: a cup of cocoa, some biscuits, and a piece of cake.

For his bravery and determination under fire, he was awarded the Military Cross. He travelled across France in an ambulance train and scrawled a letter to his mother with his left hand. He told her not to worry. He said he felt like the luckiest boy in all of France.

Banting was sent to England aboard a ship and taken to a hospital in Manchester. He spent nine weeks there while doctors debated whether to amputate his arm. He refused to let them cut it off. He was not the most sophisticated doctor around, but he was stubborn. He continued to write to his mother every Sunday.

He was released from hospital on December 4, 1918, three weeks after the conclusion of the conflict.

The war had killed and wounded millions of people. But mostly it had killed an idea, the idea that civilization was always progressing to a higher level.

In late February, 1919, Banting set sail for Canada. The ship landed in Halifax in early March. He was posted to the Christie Street Hospital in Toronto for six months, where he did orthopedic work, trying to mend the bones of wounded and crippled soldiers.

Banting was discharged from the army in the summer of 1919. He was now in his late twenties, and he hardly had any money. In the autumn of 1919 and into 1920, he was a senior house surgeon at the Hospital for Sick Children in Toronto. Edith Roach, his fiancée since 1916, had waited for him. She wanted to get married. But he wasn't earning enough money.

Banting moved to London, Ontario, and set up a medical practice. He had few patients. He hated being idle. He began to sketch pictures with pencil and paper. It occurred to him that he might sell some of his pictures.

One summer day in 1920, in London, he noticed a print for sale in the window of a store. The picture was called *The Landing*. It showed men tugging on a rope, pulling a boat up onto skids out of the water.

He went in to the store. A little bell rang on the doorframe, announcing his arrival. A salesgirl came out from the back.

"Can I help you, sir?"

"Yes, the picture in the window. How much?"

"Seventy-five cents, sir."

She wrapped the print in brown paper.

"It's pretty, isn't it," she said.

"I'd like a paintbrush, too."

"A paintbrush, sir?"

"Yes, and some paint."

"Oils or watercolours?"

"Don't know. What do you think?"

"Watercolours."

"Then I'll take watercolours."

When Banting got home he hung the print on the wall of his room. He took the cardboard backing from a laundered shirt and started to paint. He copied the print until he was satisfied with the results. He also copied pictures from old magazines and books, trying to improve his style. He thought the pictures were pretty good. He took the best ones to an art dealer in London and tried to sell them.

"You want me to buy these?" the dealer asked.

"Yes, sir, I do," Banting said.

"You must be joking."

"I wouldn't joke about a thing like this."

The dealer laughed. "You should get into some other line of work."

"What did you say?" Banting asked. His face turned red.

"No offence, mister, but I wouldn't use these pictures to line a birdcage."

"How would you like a punch in the nose," Banting said.

"There's no reason for that kind of talk," the dealer said. "Good day, sir."

Banting left the store with his paintings. He wished he had gone ahead and punched the man.

Banting was unsophisticated, and his language was coarse. He had spent most of his life as a farmhand and a soldier. His medical practice had been on the battle-field. Sometimes, a man had to use his fists.

He felt as if he had failed as a painter. But like every other failure in his life, it only made him more determined to succeed.

4

Bringing the Bones to Life

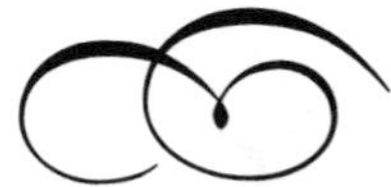

Toronto was inundated in the spring of 1922 with pleas for the miraculous substance known as insulin. Diabetic patients travelled to the city from all over North America. They were desperate. Some had only weeks to live. But now, as Macleod had predicted in Washington, there were production problems.

In March, after seven patients had been treated, the nightmare happened. J.B. Collip, the biochemist who had purified the extract, discovered he could not repeat his earlier success. He had hit upon the magic formula but had not written it down. Making insulin in 1922 was not a simple matter. He tried to produce insulin from new equipment that had been installed in

THE GIANTS - - WEEK OF JAN. 3-8, 1966

THE GIANTS
— Dr. Frederick Banting
IN MAY, 1920, A YOUNG BIOCHEMISTRY STUDENT AT THE UNIVERSITY OF TORONTO, CHARLES BEST, VOLUNTEERS TO AID DR. FREDERICK BANTING IN HIS DIABETES RESEARCH.
YOU REALIZE, MR. BEST, I CAN PAY YOU NO SALARY AND THAT MOST PEOPLE PREDICT MY EXPERIMENT WILL FAIL ?
I EXPECT NO SALARY... NOR DO I EXPECT FAILURE. IT WILL BE AN HONOR TO WORK WITH YOU, DR. BANTING.
1-3
WALT McDAYTER NORMAN DREW
EXCELLENT ! THEN WE'LL START AT ONCE. PREPARE ONE OF THE DOGS FOR SURGERY...
AND SO ON MAY 16, 1921, TWO YOUNG CANADIANS LAUNCH AN EXPERIMENT THAT WILL AFFECT MILLIONS OF LIVES THE WORLD OVER !
THE GIANTS
— Dr. Frederick Banting
DR. FREDERICK BANTING AND CHARLES BEST PERFORM TWO TYPES OF SURGERY ON THEIR DOGS : IN ONE GROUP THEY INDUCE DIABETES, IN THE OTHER THEY BLOCK THE PANCREAS TO ISOLATE A HORMONE CALLED ISLETIN.
WALT McDAYTER NORMAN DREW
SOON THEY'VE EXTRACTED A SAMPLE OF THIS ISLETIN (THE HORMONE WE NOW KNOW AS INSULIN).
NEXT STEP... TO INJECT THIS INTO ONE OF THE DOGS WITH DIABETES.
IF OUR THEORY'S RIGHT, THIS INJECTION WILL COMBAT THE DISEASE IN THE DOG.
1-4
AND SO ON JULY 27, 1921, FOR THE FIRST TIME PURE INSULIN IS TESTED... IN AN EXPERIMENT WHICH WILL BE BOTH A SUCCESS AND A FAILURE !
THE GIANTS
— Dr. Frederick Banting
DR. FREDERICK BANTING AND CHARLES BEST ARE ELATED OVER IMMEDIATE RESULTS FOLLOWING THEIR INJECTION OF ISLETIN (INSULIN) INTO A DIABETIC DOG.
YESTERDAY THIS DOG WAS DYING... NOW HE'S AS PERKY AS A PUP !
UNFORTUNATELY, THOUGH THEY PROVE THEIR POINT, THEY LOSE THEIR PATIENT. NEXT DAY, THE DOG IS DEAD !
1-5
BUT I DON'T UNDERSTAND, DR. BANTING. THE DOG SEEMED SO HEALTHY, CURED OF DIABETES...
WALT McDAYTER NORMAN DREW
NO, NOT CURED, BUT OUR ISLETIN DID CONTROL THE DIABETES. THIS MEANS WE CAN HELP DIABETICS ONLY IF THEY CONTINUALLY TAKE INJECTIONS.
BUT IS THERE A SOURCE OF ISLETIN SOMEWHERE SO GREAT THAT IT WILL SUPPLY EVERY DIABETIC IN THE WORLD WITH INJECTIONS EVERY DAY OF HIS LIFE ?

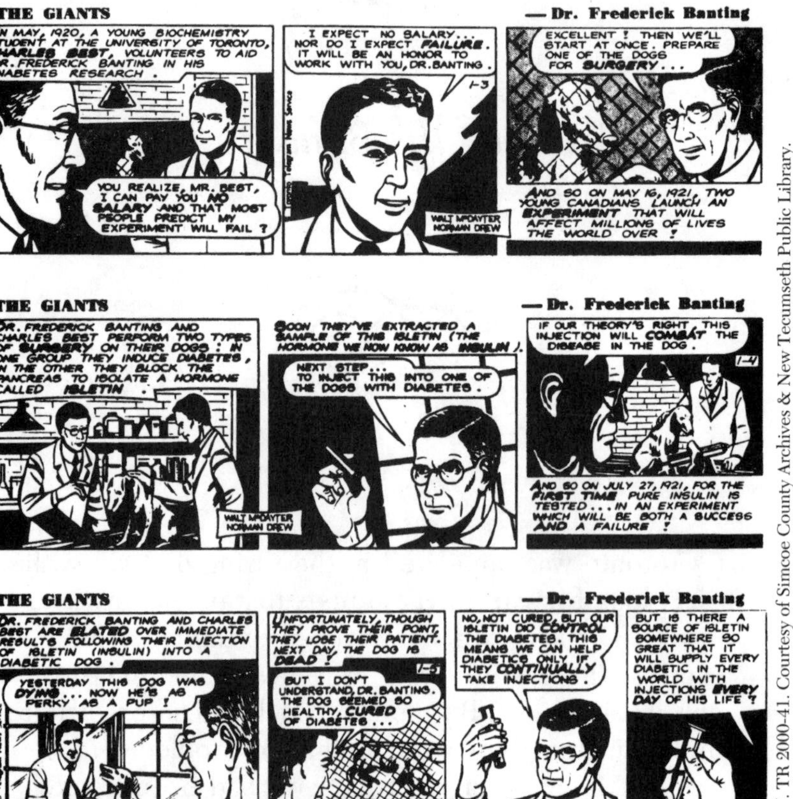

10007. TR 2000-41. Courtesy of Simcoe County Archives & New Tecumseth Public Library.

The public view of Banting, the Great Man who discovered insulin.

the Medical Building, but the batches for some reason were weak. When he tried to produce insulin on a small scale in the laboratory, he got the same poor results.

Banting, Best, and Macleod worked to rediscover the extract, but without success. One of the severely diabetic patients, a little girl, went into a coma. They brought her back to life with the inferior insulin, but when it ran out, she died. They found themselves in the middle of an insulin famine. Banting was furious with Collip. The problems with Macleod, the feeling of being shut out of his own discovery, the girl who died. Banting began to drink heavily again.

Late one March night, Best went to Banting's Grenville Street room.

When he opened the door, the thick, bluish smoke from Banting's pipe rolled into the hall. Banting was seated at a small table with a glass of lab alcohol in one hand and his pipe in the other. He was unshaven, and his hair looked as if it hadn't seen a brush in days. His eyes were bloodshot.

"Don't just stand there, Charley, come in."

"You look like hell," Best said.

"I can't do it anymore," Banting said. "I quit."

"You can't quit."

"Macleod and Collip. They let us down." Tears came to Banting's eyes. "That little girl," he said. "The one who died. Jesus." His hand tightened around the glass. "I want to go somewhere I can think in peace. Where my work is respected. There's the States. I could go there."

"We belong here," Best said. "But if you go, I go with you. We're in this together."

"Do you mean it?"

"You bet I do."

The expression of loyalty was just what Banting needed to hear. He knocked his drink back, and set the glass on the table.

"There's work to do, Charley," Banting said. "I'm not going to touch another drop of alcohol until insulin is saving diabetics."

"It's a deal," Best said. They shook hands, and wiped the table clean. With pencil and paper they began planning the next crucial steps in the development of insulin.

Less than two months later, Best, working with Banting, produced the first potent extract the group had seen in a long time. He gave his batch to Banting, who had already opened a medical office on Bloor Street West. The Christie Street Military Hospital also opened a diabetes clinic. The Christie Street patients were made available to Banting, who still did not have clinical privileges at Toronto General Hospital.

The first patient to receive the newer, potent extract was Joe Gilchrist, Banting's medical school buddy who had volunteered to swallow "isletin" six months before, demonstrating that the extract had no effect when taken orally. Gilchrist began using insulin. He also began working with Banting at the Christie Street clinic.

Toward the end of May, Banting gave a batch of insulin to an American physician, Dr. John Williams of Rochester, New York, just across Lake Ontario from Toronto. Dr. Williams was trying to save the life of a twenty-two-year-old diabetic patient named James

Havens, the son of a vice-president of Eastman-Kodak, the film and camera company. Havens was the first American resident to receive insulin.

To his dismay, Dr. Williams found that the insulin had no effect on his patient. Banting rushed to Rochester and advised him to increase the dose. It worked, and the patient improved dramatically. Banting warned Dr. Williams against any publicity, because there wasn't enough insulin to go around.

Best was placed in charge of insulin production at the Connaught Lab. It was agreed that two-thirds of Connaught's insulin production would go to Banting, to be split between his private practice and the Christie Street clinic. The remaining one-third was for Toronto General Hospital and the Hospital for Sick Children.

Banting had discovered insulin at the University of Toronto. His appointment in the university's pharmacology department, which allowed him to continue his research, had expired. Yet, even after insulin had been discovered, the university denied him an appointment in the department of medicine and in the school's teaching hospital, Toronto General. The basis of the decision was that Banting did not have the proper qualifications, since he was not actually practising medicine. The real problem may have been that the two-fisted Banting upset the conservative, academic medical establishment in Toronto. He was looked upon as wild, impulsive, and temperamental.

Banting may not have been Toronto's cup of tea, but he was starting to get offers to leave Canada and work in the United States.

Banting, Macleod, and the others accepted a proposal from the Eli Lilly and Company to collaborate in the development of insulin. Based in Indianapolis, Indiana, Lilly was a respected, family-owned drug company that sold only to doctors and pharmacists. It had a modern research facility. The agreement between the Board of Governors of the University of Toronto and Eli Lilly and Company limited the company's sales to the United States and the Americas. Toronto was to receive royalties from sales to support research.

In June, Best and Collip travelled to Indianapolis and told the Lilly chemists all they knew about producing insulin. They helped with the first attempt to produce the extract. After that, Collip returned to his job at the University of Alberta.

During the summer of 1922, Connaught was trying to produce enough insulin for Canada. However, production had all but stopped, and the quality of the insulin was poor because the equipment was inadequate.

Banting wanted Toronto to have the same kind of modern equipment that Eli Lilly had in Indianapolis and went to see the chairman of the university's board of governors. The situation was urgent. Lives were at stake. But he was told it was impossible to get the money for new equipment until the board had its next formal meeting, when the proposal would be discussed. Banting was outraged at this attitude, which he found typical of bureaucrats in Canada. He remembered a doctor in New York who had promised him money for research. He took the train to New York City and asked the doctor for help. The doctor phoned a wealthy friend who had a very sick diabetic child. After a few minutes Banting had the money for equipment to produce potent insulin, and the doctor had insulin for his friend's child.

In the summer of 1922, the chairman of Toronto General Hospital's board of trustees, C.S. Blackwell, was visiting American hospitals. It was then he realized the importance of what Banting had done. Insulin was big, very big. He cut off his trip, returned to Toronto, and saw about getting Banting clinical privileges at the hospital so he could start treating diabetics.

Also that summer, an American financier showed up at Banting's boarding house room and offered him $1 million in cash and 5 per cent of insulin royalties if he would only hand over the patents to a group on Wall Street. The American looked around at Banting's smoke-filled room, more of a cubicle, really. He eyed the lone table and chair and wondered why the doctor was living like that when he could have it all, the big house in the country, the big car, the servants.

"I can promise you," the man said, "that a chain of clinics will be established across the United States and Canada with you as medical director. The only patients you'll ever have to see will be wealthy. You will be set for life. You can't lose, doctor."

"No, thanks," Banting said.

Two nights later, the man phoned him from New York and repeated the offer. Banting again said no.

Later, whenever Banting told the story, he would always refuse to identify the financier.

In August, clinical trials of insulin began in the United States with two of the world's most famous diabetologists, Dr. Elliott Joslin of Boston, Massachusetts and Dr. Frederick Allen of Morristown, New Jersey. Allen was the originator of the "undernutrition therapy" Banting had been taught in medical school. At the Physiatric Institute, Allen's diabetic clinic, rumours began to spread that something important was going to happen. Normally, the patients had no hope of survival. They knew that diabetes was a death sentence. To control their blood sugar, and gain a few months of life, they were kept on starvation diets. They ate bread husks and boiled fruit. Their bones stuck out; their faces were like skulls. They looked like living corpses.

All patients were required to go to bed after the evening meal. One evening, they were told that Dr. Allen had something to tell them. About fifty men and women in various stages of starvation stirred from their beds and began walking to the foyer of the building. They were skin and bone. Some of them clung to the walls for support, moving slowly, tenderly, as if they had just been resurrected from the dead and were getting to know mortality again. When they had assembled in one place, they cast their eyes to the floor. They didn't know what to expect. Dr. Allen's steps, and his wife's steps, could be heard outside as they approached the building. The doctor walked briskly down the hall and stood in front of his patients. For a few moments, he could not speak.

"I have some good news for you," he said. "An extract has been discovered in Toronto that can be used in the treatment of diabetes. This I can tell you: it is saving the lives of diabetics right now. With this extract, called insulin, diabetics can lead normal lives."

There was silence. No one moved. But on some of the faces, tears began to fall.

Dr. Allen administered insulin to six of his most critically ill patients. He injected small amounts, one-half unit per injection, to conserve the supply. The results were miraculous.

Dr. Joslin saw the same awesome effects on his patients, even patients who had gone into a diabetic coma. They awakened. Their vigour returned, their eyes grew bright, and their skin began to glow. They lost their profound mental depression. They gained weight and became cheerful again and interested in life. He felt he was witnessing the resurrection of the dead.

In an address Joslin delivered in 1934 at the opening of new research laboratories at Eli Lilly, he said Banting's discovery reminded him of the thirty-seventh chapter of the Book of Ezekiel. He said he called this chapter, the "Banting" chapter. When the word came from Toronto in 1922 that insulin had been discovered, he said, he thought of the prophetic words in Ezekiel 37:1-10.

The hand of the Lord was upon me, and carried me out in the spirit of the Lord, and set me down in the midst of the valley which was full of bones, and caused me to pass by them round about: and, behold, there were very many in the open valley; and, lo, they were very dry.

And he said unto me, "Son of man, can these bones live?" And I answered, "O Lord God, thou knowest." Again he said unto me, "Prophesy upon these bones, and say unto them, 'O ye dry bones, hear the word of the Lord. Thus saith the Lord God unto these bones; Behold, I will cause breath to enter into you, and ye shall live: And I will lay sinews upon you, and will bring up flesh upon you, and cover you with skin, and put breath in you, and ye shall live; and ye shall know that I am the Lord.'" So I prophesied as I was commanded: and as I prophesied, there was a noise, and behold a shaking, and the bones came together, bone to his bone.

And when I beheld, lo, the sinews and the flesh came up upon them, and the skin covered them above: but there was no breath in them.

Then he said unto me, "Prophesy unto the wind, prophesy, son of man, and say to the wind, 'Thus saith the Lord God: Come from the four winds, O breath, and breathe upon these slain, that they may live.'"

So I prophesied as he commanded me, and the breath came into them, and they lived, and stood up upon their feet, an exceeding great army.

The diabetic clinic at Toronto General Hospital, with Banting as an attending physician, opened its doors on August 21, 1922. Most of the diabetics in the hospital were being injected with insulin produced by Eli Lilly, but the Connaught Lab, with new equipment that Banting had purchased with American money when the Canadians wouldn't come forward, soon began producing potent insulin too.

In Toronto and Boston, in other cities, and eventually in Europe and the rest of the world, diabetics were waking up from the long sleep of the living dead.

The discovery of insulin transferred the responsibility of the diabetic's life from the doctor to the patient. Diabetics could administer their own injections. Once upon a time, doctors could only hope to extend the life of a diabetic by a few months, perhaps a year or two. Insulin had changed that.

Banting's idea to ligate the ducts of dog pancreases was unimportant from a technical standpoint. Through trial and error, he eventually abandoned his original plan. He finally hit upon the idea that an extract could be produced from whole beef pancreas. But that was how artists and scientists had always worked. The first pages of a book or the first steps of an experiment were often subject to transformation. The idea that Banting had in London in 1920 was a brilliant stroke of the imagination that started him down the road of discovery. His first experiments in dramatically lowering the blood sugar of dogs, and in keeping diabetic dogs alive with this primitive extract, were good enough to convince Macleod to move ahead with the research. Banting's inexperience, his relative lack of knowledge about diabetes, helped him because it allowed his imagination to roam.

Insulin began with Banting and became his life. It emerged in 1921-22 as the result of a collaboration by all four researchers: Banting, Best, Collip, and

Macleod. But it was almost as if Banting, single-handed, had wrestled the insulin problem to the ground on those first sweltering nights in Toronto, when his idea was still not being taken seriously by the experts.

As the principal discoverer of insulin, Banting would be showered with awards, money, and unending gratitude. No single event in the history of medicine had changed the lives of so many people, so suddenly. Banting, a twenty-nine-year-old farmer's son who had barely attracted a handful of patients as a physician, had succeeded where so many great scientists had failed.

As the summer was ending, Collip was in Alberta, Macleod was in New Brunswick studying the properties of fish pancreas, and Best was vacationing in Maine. Banting was in Toronto, about to meet one of his most famous patients, fourteen-year-old Elizabeth Hughes.

Elizabeth Hughes was the daughter of Charles Evans Hughes, a former U.S. presidential candidate now serving as Secretary of State in the administration of President Warren Harding. The little girl had been diagnosed with diabetes in 1919. In 1922 she was only 1.5 metres tall and weighed about twenty kilograms. She had been rigidly following the Allen "starvation" diet. Her brittle hair was falling out. She looked like a tiny skeleton and had kept herself alive through sheer determination.

In August her mother brought her to Toronto. She responded immediately to Banting's injections of insulin. The sugar disappeared from her urine and her blood sugar dropped to normal. Banting knew virtually nothing about diabetes treatment or the principles of dietary adjustment. He had only six months' experience treating diabetics. As an old-fashioned physician, he used his common sense. What a young, bone-thin girl really needed was to eat good food and gain some weight. He put Elizabeth on a normal diet with lots of butter and cream. He didn't want anyone to know he was breaking the rules and made her Joslin-trained private nurse promise not to tell. Elizabeth began to grow taller. She gained weight, a kilogram each week. She could not believe how her life had changed with insulin. She had been on the verge of death, and now she was alive, enthusiastic, happy. She adored Banting and got to see his office and the room where he lived. She saw the pictures he had painted in his spare time and the detective novels he liked to read. She thought he was a great doctor, and a great artist, too.

In November, 1922, a group of American diabetologists, including Elliott Joslin and Frederick Allen, came to Toronto for three days' discussion of insulin. Both Joslin and Allen had been treating Elizabeth, and they were looking forward to seeing her again. The last time they saw her, she was emaciated. Her muscles were wasted, her shoulders drooped, and her abdomen protruded from severe malnutrition. She could barely walk. She had been depressed, which was only natural considering she had been waiting to die.

For three months, she had been in Dr. Banting's care. She had been receiving daily insulin injections. The extract still sometimes contained impurities. Weak insulin had to be taken in frequent, larger doses, and often left abscesses or swelling at the sites of the injections. But she was alive. She was thriving. On the last day of the three-day conference, Banting showed her off to the doctors. When they walked into the room, they did not recognize her.

"Gentlemen," Dr. Banting said. "I'd like you to meet Elizabeth Hughes."

"Oh!" Dr. Allen said. "Oh!"

Dr. Joslin stared, mouth open.

Standing before them was a lovely young girl with satiny hair, bright eyes, and a smile that could melt ice cream.

She had filled out so much, new links had to be added to her favourite bracelet.

She smiled at the doctors.

Awestruck, they said hello.

"I've never seen anything like it," Dr. Allen said.

The girl who had been nothing but bones, who had been waiting in death's cold anteroom, ready to leave this world, was healthy. The last time they saw her, she had been an invalid. Her main activities had been sewing and reading in bed. Now she was going to concerts and movies and to the park. She toured the Connaught laboratory in the basement of the Medical Building and saw how insulin was produced in day and night shifts. She was eating bread and mashed potatoes swimming in butter, foods that had once been forbidden. Best of all, whenever she had a hypoglycemic reaction from the insulin, and her blood sugar plummeted, Dr. Banting gave her molasses candy kisses.

❧

By that fall, insulin was starting to be used clinically across North America. Wherever Banting spoke, at a luncheon of dignitaries in Toronto or an audience of medical students at Harvard, he was greeted with a standing ovation.

In February, 1923, Banting and Best returned to Banting's hometown of Alliston. A public reception was held in the town hall. After a round of community singing, Best stood up and outlined the details of the discovery. Then it was Banting's turn. His parents, Margaret and William, were on stage with him.

"It would have been impossible to do my research without the support of these two people," he said, turning to them. The crowd erupted in applause.

When the hall had quieted down, he told the young people of Alliston to work hard if they wanted to succeed. His parents, by example, had taught him that.

But he had also learned about hard work from the books his father read to the family in the kitchen. *The Pilgrim's Progress*, which was used as a companion to the Bible, emphasized activity, sweat, and struggle. There was no such thing as divine intervention for the lazy. The hero, Christian, had to keep knocking on the gates before they were opened. The same could be said for Banting and the discovery of insulin. The idea came quietly in the night, but without the work, and the struggle, it was nothing.

When reporters rushed up to Banting's mother after the speech and asked about her son, she told them she still remembered him as the little boy who used to put his arm around her waist while she gathered eggs in the henhouse. He was still his mother's son.

5

The Nobel Prize

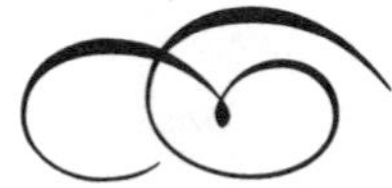

In 1923, Fred Banting was the most famous man in Canada. He was thirty-two years old and looking for a wife. He began dating some of the nurses from Toronto General Hospital. It wasn't hard for him to get a date. The nurses were knocking on his door.

He was attracted to Marion Robertson, the tall, fair-haired daughter of a doctor from the nearby town of Elora, Ontario. Marion was an X-ray technician at the hospital and was well-connected socially. But Fred was still engaged to Edith Roach. He had his fame to deal with. He was a busy man.

Every week he got letters and gifts from grateful diabetics all over the world. Total strangers came up to

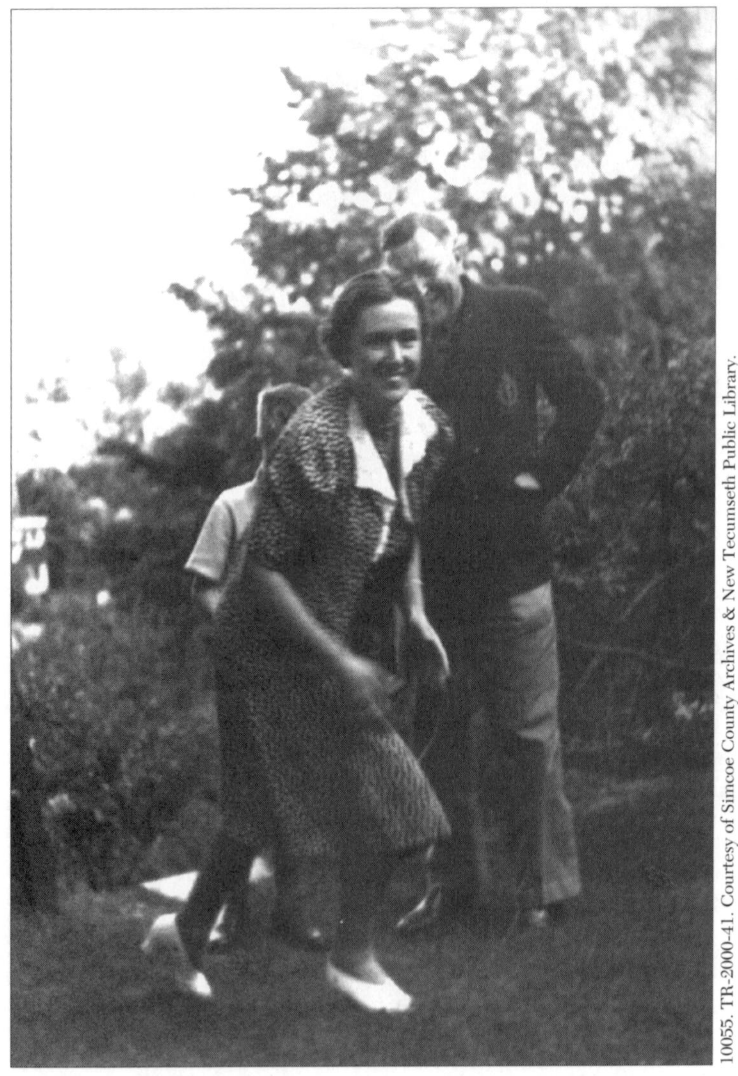

10055. TR-2000-41. Courtesy of Simcoe County Archives & New Tecumseth Public Library.

Banting and his first wife, Marion, in happier days
when their marriage was strong.

him on the street and shook his hand and thanked him for what he had done.

In the summer of 1923, Banting was en route to England on the *Empress of France* for a round of conferences and sightseeing. It was his first trip to Europe since the Great War. Cables and letters of congratulations and praise followed him across the ocean. Walking the deck of the liner, he looked out at the rolling sea. He could see only good fortune ahead.

The Ontario government announced it would establish the Banting and Best Chair of Medical Research at the University of Toronto, funded with an annual grant of $10,000. Banting was named permanent Professor of Medical Research, with an annual salary of $5,000. In June, 1923, the Canadian House of Commons unanimously voted to grant Banting, in recognition of the discovery of insulin, a lifetime annuity of $7,500, a substantial sum of money in those days – enough to allow him to devote his life to medical research.

Three years before, Banting was a physician with no research training to speak of and few prospects. He was lucky to make more than a few dollars a month. Now he was making at least $12,500 a year, with a lifetime appointment to do any research he liked.

Macleod, Best, and Collip were not being recognized in Canada for their part in the discovery of insulin. The money earmarked for Banting was for him alone. Best complained that he had not even been mentioned in the annuity granted by the House of Commons. There was nothing Banting could do. He wrote Best, saying he wished the government would give him an equal amount.

All Banting wanted now was to work in a lab on new ideas, without interruption. He was growing sick and tired of the fame that insulin had brought.

At luncheons and dinners, in hospitals and labs, he was being introduced to all the leading medical and scientific experts in Europe. For Banting, it was an ordeal. He listened to discussions on biochemistry, music, theatre, literature, art, and politics. He made up his mind to devote some time each day to subjects outside the field of medicine so that he could hold his own with people of culture.

In London, Banting was invited to meet King George V. He was to appear at Buckingham Palace at ten in the morning, July 18. He shopped for a silk hat, gloves, and all the required items of dress.

When he arrived at the Palace he was taken upstairs along a wide corridor, into a room with a table at the centre. His collar was tight and his new shoes squeaked when he walked. He began to sweat. He felt like a farmboy.

Finally, he was announced. He was left alone with the King, who wanted to know all about the discovery of insulin. At first, Banting didn't like being alone with the King. He was afraid if something happened to His Majesty, he would be blamed. But he soon felt at ease.

"Come over here," the King said. "To the window."

They looked out over the palace grounds. A groundskeeper was pushing a wheelbarrow.

"See that man down there?" the King said. "He is a diabetic. People from all walks of life, including some of my acquaintances, owe their lives to you and your colleagues in Canada. Is it true what they say about insulin, that it has resurrected the dead?"

"The patients were dead, in a sense," Banting replied. "In cases where the patient has been in a coma, and believed dead, the patient has found life again. But there is another kind of resurrection. I remember one case in particular. Would you like to hear it?"

"I certainly would."

"It was last summer, when the extract was precious and hard to come by. I was sitting in my office when a man carried his wife into the room. He was a handsome man in his thirties. He deposited his wife in an easy chair. She weighed about thirty or thirty-five kilograms. Her eyes were almost shut with edema, her skin was hard, like parchment, and her red hair was so thin you could see her scalp. Her ankles were swollen, and her skin had sores where they stretched over the bones. I felt sorry for the husband. She snarled at him and bossed him around. The man was like a slave to her foul disposition."

The King laughed. "Even a king must be a slave once in a while."

"Still, I could not understand why he took it patiently. I placed her in hospital, but she was an uncooperative patient. She scolded him. Cursed him. He wasn't permitted to leave the hospital at night until she was asleep. She received insulin in hospital, and when she improved was sent home and told to continue her injections."

Banting said he did not write to them, or follow up. Months later, he said, he was at his desk when his office door was thrown open and in rushed one of the most beautiful women he had ever seen. He was sure he had never seen her before. He told her he didn't think they had been introduced, but she threw her arms around his neck and kissed him. Over her head he spotted the laughing face of the patient husband.

"We stood there, hand in hand," Banting continued. "The husband said he wanted me to see his wife the way she was now, the way she was before they married, before she had diabetes.

"Months later I received an envelope with a pink ribbon in it and the name of their baby daughter. I wondered if she had red hair, like her mother, and I prayed she would never have diabetes."

"That is my prayer, too," the King said. "But even if she does, you have made it possible for her to have a wonderful life."

He wished Banting well.

On his way out of the Palace the famous physician was surrounded by journalists.

"Where's Dr. Banting?"

"What did the King say?"

"Did they talk about ice hockey? An anecdote, a joke. Give us something, will you?"

"When is Banting coming out?"

"Pretty soon," Banting remarked.

He jumped into a waiting cab.

It wasn't until the car pulled away that the reporters realized who he was. They ran after him, shouting, waving their arms. The car disappeared into the traffic. Banting was the elusive Canadian, the homespun genius who couldn't be bothered with the mighty press. Now the reporters wanted him more than ever. But Banting hated talking to the press. Reporters never seemed to get his quotes right, and once his mangled comments were in the paper there was nothing he could do about it. The news media had helped spread Banting's fame, but he wished the reporters would leave him alone.

His first medical talk in Britain was before an international congress of surgeons in London. He had always dreaded public speaking. He delivered an almost inaudible two-minute speech on the discovery of insulin. In Edinburgh, on July 24, at the Eleventh International Physiological Congress, Banting was more relaxed as he gave several short papers on insulin experiments.

Macleod was in Edinburgh, too. He gave the keynote address on insulin at one of the general sessions. He thanked the congress on behalf of himself and his collaborators.

Attending the insulin sessions was a group from the Caroline Institute in Stockholm, Sweden. Members of the institute's Nobel committee were there to determine whether the discovery of insulin was worthy of the Nobel Prize.

(Nominations for the Nobel Prize in Physiology or Medicine arrived at the institute in December 1922 and January 1923. Banting and Macleod were nominated separately. But August Krogh, a Danish physiologist and Nobel Laureate who was working on insulin, nominated both Banting and Macleod. The Nobel committee was allowed to award the prize to one person, but not more than three. Krogh nominated the two men not only for the discovery of insulin, but also for the exploration of its practical application in clinical use.)

Banting's ship docked at Quebec on August 18. He hid from reporters and when they finally caught up with him he wondered why they couldn't just leave him in peace.

He was persuaded to open the Canadian National Exhibition (CNE) in Toronto, on August 25. He issued a plea for more support for medical research to keep talented Canadians in the country. The special medals for achievers at the 1923 CNE had a likeness of Banting on one side. His mother and father were also at the exhibition. His mother was asked if she were proud of her son. "Not proud, thankful," she replied. She bought a new pair of thin black gloves for the occasion. By the time the exhibition was over, the gloves were worn through from all the handshaking.

Finally, in the fall of 1923, Banting settled down to work in his laboratory in Toronto.

On October 26, after spending the day with his parents on the farm, Banting drove back to Toronto. The phone rang in his office. A friend was on the line.

"Fred, have you heard?"

"What?"

"Haven't you seen the papers?"

"No."

"You and Macleod were awarded the Nobel Prize!"

"Go to hell," he said, and hung up.

Banting was in no mood for practical jokes. He just wanted to work. A newspaper was in the office. He picked it up and looked at the front page. There it was.

Frederick G. Banting and J.J.R. Macleod had been awarded the Nobel Prize in Medicine for the discovery of insulin. Banting exploded. There was no mention of Best. It was Macleod! Macleod would share the glory.

He threw down the paper, got in his car, and sped to his laboratory. He was going to confront Macleod. But going up the steps into the building he met a friend, J.G. Fitzgerald, the head of Connaught Laboratories, which was producing insulin for the Canadian market. Banting told him he was going to refuse the prize and that the Nobel people in Stockholm could all go to hell in a handbasket. He asked Fitzgerald to name one idea in the insulin research that was Macleod's, or one experiment that he had done with his own hands. Fitzgerald took Banting by the arm and asked him to speak to Colonel Albert Gooderham, a member of the university's board of governors and one of the few men Banting trusted.

After congratulating him, Gooderham told Banting to cool down. He reminded him that he was the first Canadian to win the Nobel Prize. (Macleod was a native of Scotland.) He asked Banting to think of his country. What would people say if he turned down the Nobel Prize? What would the world think? Banting calmed down.

He decided to share his prize with Best, who was in Massachusetts to address students at Harvard Medical School. After Best finished his talk, Dr. Elliott Joslin, the famous American diabetologist, got up and read a telegram from Banting: "... I ascribe to Best equal share in the discovery (stop) hurt that he not so acknowledged by Nobel trustees (stop) will share with him."

Macleod announced a few days later that he would share his half of the prize with Collip. Macleod told the press that Collip had an equal share in the discovery, but had to issue a clarification a few days later saying he was entitled to a "fair share" of the credit. Banting and Macleod would share the $40,000 ($30,000 Canadian) prize money with Best and Collip. Banting's one-quarter share was $7,750, a princely sum compared to his four-dollar-a month days.

(Voting by secret ballot, the nineteen assembled professors of the Caroline Institute awarded the 1923 Nobel Prize in Medicine to Banting because of his idea and initiative, and Macleod because he had guided the scientific work to a conclusion.)

On November 26, the University of Toronto awarded honorary Doctor of Science degrees to both its Nobel laureates. Banting gave a speech in which he spoke well of Macleod.

It appeared the bad feelings had gone. But under the surface, the bitterness simmered.

Banting's personal life was in turmoil. He and Edith signed an agreement in May 1924, in which she gave up all claims on him in return for $2,000 and the return of her ring that he sometimes wore around his key chain. They had met thirteen years ago. Her relationship with Fred had moments of happiness, but those moments weren't enough to keep it alive.

Edith eventually married, but she never had children.

In the summer of 1924, Banting was pursuing the beautiful Marion Robertson. He also was spending long hours in the lab, operating on dogs and trying to isolate the hormones of the adrenal cortex in a search for the "elixir of life."

He and Marion decided to marry, but their plans were almost scuttled by a letter that could have been written for a radio soap opera.

An unsigned typewritten letter was mailed to Marion that warned her not to marry Fred. The letter suggested he was a "cad," a schemer, a man who exploits women. The letter writer said her life had been ruined, and that if Banting ever got married she planned to sue him for breach of promise, evidently the promise of marriage he had made. Marion may have received the letter the day it was mailed. It was not from Edith. It may have been from a woman Banting had been dating, someone who felt that he had backed out of a marriage proposal.

The letter had no apparent effect on the sweethearts. On June 4, 1924, Fred and Marion were married in the home of Marion's uncle, with only the immediate families in attendance. Some of the Philathea Bible class girls who had known Banting when he was struggling to find insulin, the ones who brought him meals while he worked in his lab, found out about the event and gathered outside to blow kisses and congratulate their hero when he came down the steps with his bride.

The Bantings spent a few days at the Preston Springs Hotel, about one hundred kilometres west of Toronto. But they were soon off to the eastern United

States. Fred received an honorary degree from Yale University for service to humanity "beyond all measure," and gave a paper on diabetes in the resort town of Atlantic City, New Jersey. He and his wife strolled the wide sandy beaches and watched the moon shine on the waves, and it seemed as if their happiness would never end.

In mid-July they went on their real honeymoon, a medical junket in the Caribbean sponsored by the United Fruit Company, a U.S.-based multinational corporation with extensive holdings in the tropics. The two-month trip would take them to Cuba, Jamaica, and Central and South America. They would return to New York in September.

Banting and other prominent medical men from around the world attended the ten-day, expense-paid conference on health problems in Latin America. The conference was at the Myrtle Bank Hotel in Kingston, Jamaica. The physicians learned about tropical diseases and toured hospitals, universities, and a leper colony.

Banting was worried about his paper on "Insulin in the Treatment of Diabetes." While Marion danced, he walked down the lawn of the hotel to the beach and read the paper to another doctor beneath the electric lights and the palm trees. He was always concerned that his papers might not be good enough. Perhaps he couldn't forget the embarrassment he felt as a schoolboy when he failed his compositions and spelling tests. But his paper on insulin and diabetes was a success.

He wondered why he was at the conference. Diabetes was not a tropical disease, and it was not contagious. It was clear that he was asked to attend because he was a Nobel laureate, the discoverer of insulin, one of the most famous men in the world.

On one of his tours Banting observed that natives who ate raw sugar cane apparently did not have a propensity to diabetes. He toyed with the idea that consumption of refined white sugar might lead to the disease, but he never came to any firm conclusions.

For Marion, the trip was one glorious social event. She met famous people and went to parties. Banting rarely had the opportunity to relax. He read detective stories and smoked his pipe but spent most of his time writing and delivering papers and touring tropical medical facilities.

Banting's biggest realization at the conference had nothing to do with medicine. It had to do with his marriage. It was clear that it wasn't working, and that he and Marion had few common interests. For his vivacious young bride, the trip was wonderful: dancing, moonlit nights, and parties. For the rough doctor, who despised small talk and socializing, the trip was a cruise right out of hell, the voyage of the damned.

During the day, Banting toured hospitals and clinics and saw people with gruesome tropical diseases. He wanted to unwind in the evening with Marion. He expected her to be the dutiful bride and to want what he wanted. They spent a few quiet evenings together but began to argue. He did not like to dance, and he often found himself sitting in a corner while his wife danced with someone else.

Their differences were highlighted on the Cuban leg of the trip. Only about 150 kilometres off the Florida coast, Cuba had become a playground for fashionable Americans, bootleggers and gamblers. The Ward Line and the United Fruit Company, Banting's sponsor for the trip, had built luxurious passenger ships to handle the booming tourist trade. Sugar was Cuba's main cash crop, and the lucrative sugar industry was largely in the hands of American companies. It appeared that Cuba was a paradise. But the economy, based on the fluctuating sugar market, was in shambles.

When the Bantings arrived in Havana, they saw, against a backdrop of blue sky, bougainvillea, and royal palms that swayed in the breeze, a city in chaos. The ill and indigent lay in the street without food or medical care. Children stood in front of marble villas begging for food while limousines glided by: Rolls-Royces, Hispano-Suizas, Cadillacs. The people who lived in the villas did not have to worry. Their houses were protected by tall iron fences with razor-sharp railings.

Cuba's leading yellow fever specialist, Dr. Aristides Agramonte, took the Bantings on a tour of Havana in an open car driven by a liveried Spanish chauffeur. That night, in their hotel, the Bantings dressed for dinner and talked about their day.

"Wasn't Dr. Agramonte's touring car just grand?" Marion said. "What a beautiful colour, dark red."

"The car was comfortable enough," Banting said. "Can't say much for the Cubans."

"I thought Dr. Agramonte was a perfect gentleman." She walked over to the window, brushing her hair. Lights glittered in the harbour.

"The hospital I saw had a thousand beds," Banting remarked. He frowned. He couldn't tie his bow tie.

"I liked it when we went to his villa afterwards and had refreshments in the courtyard," Marion said. "What was the name of that cocktail?"

"He took me to see a monument to Cuban medical students who were shot by the Spanish in 1871 – awful."

"Fred, don't always dwell on the negative."

"Did you see the Cubans sleeping on the street? There are only two classes in Cuba – rich and poor. The wealthy women grow fat in their rocking chairs, and the poor people live in congested little shacks with their laundry hanging everywhere."

"You spoke splendidly about insulin yesterday. They admire you. After your speech, did you try the champagne punch?"

"No, I had one of the sandwiches. I don't care that much for the food."

"I loved the drive we took in the moonlight. The chauffeur didn't say a word."

"It was late. I was tired."

"And then dancing on the roof garden of the Seville Hotel! Havana is a fairyland. I wish we could stay here forever."

"I just wish we didn't have to go out tonight. We could stay in. The two of us."

"But that would be impossible."

"Impossible," Banting said. "Always impossible."

In September the Bantings returned to Toronto. They had a three-storey brick and sandstone home built at

46 Bedford Road, north of the university. It was a beautiful home, tastefully furnished. Their first houseguest was Lord Dawson of Penn, physician to the King.

But for all its beauty, the home was not warm. Fred and Marion continued to grow apart.

In August, 1925, the Bantings sailed from Quebec for Europe on the *Empress of Scotland*. Marion could not believe the luxury. A maid drew her bath and called her when it was ready. The maid also brought them tea before they were up in the morning, and laid out their dinner clothes in the evening. Fred had an English valet who hardly spoke a word and always seemed to anticipate his every need. Fred and Marion were living in a fairy tale where wishes come true the moment you make them.

Their destination was Stockholm, where Banting was to give his Nobel address for the prize that was awarded two years earlier.

The speech he gave was humble and direct. It began: "I very deeply appreciate the honour which you have conferred upon me in awarding the Nobel Prize for 1923 to me and Professor J.J.R. Macleod. I am fully aware of the responsibility which rests upon me to deliver an address in which certain aspects of the work on insulin may be placed before you. This I propose to do tonight and I regret that an earlier opportunity has not been afforded me of satisfying this obligation."

Everywhere he went in Sweden, he was showered with presents and flowers by grateful diabetics. That was more important to him than all the awards in the world.

6

Waiting for Another Great Idea

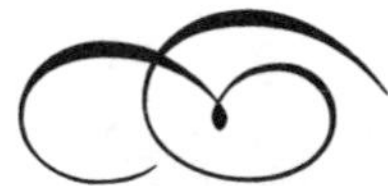

Banting wanted to find the "elixir of life." He wanted to find the place in the body where antitoxins, substances that prevent infection, are formed. He believed he could isolate these antitoxins in the adrenal cortex, the outer layer of the adrenal glands, above the kidneys. The adrenal glands produce hormones that influence vital functions of the body. Newspapers picked up the story that Banting was on the track of something "better" than insulin.

His new home was only a short distance from his lab on University Avenue. There he experimented on dogs, removing their adrenal glands and trying to keep them alive with an extract made from fresh cortex. By

Banting House, London, Ontario

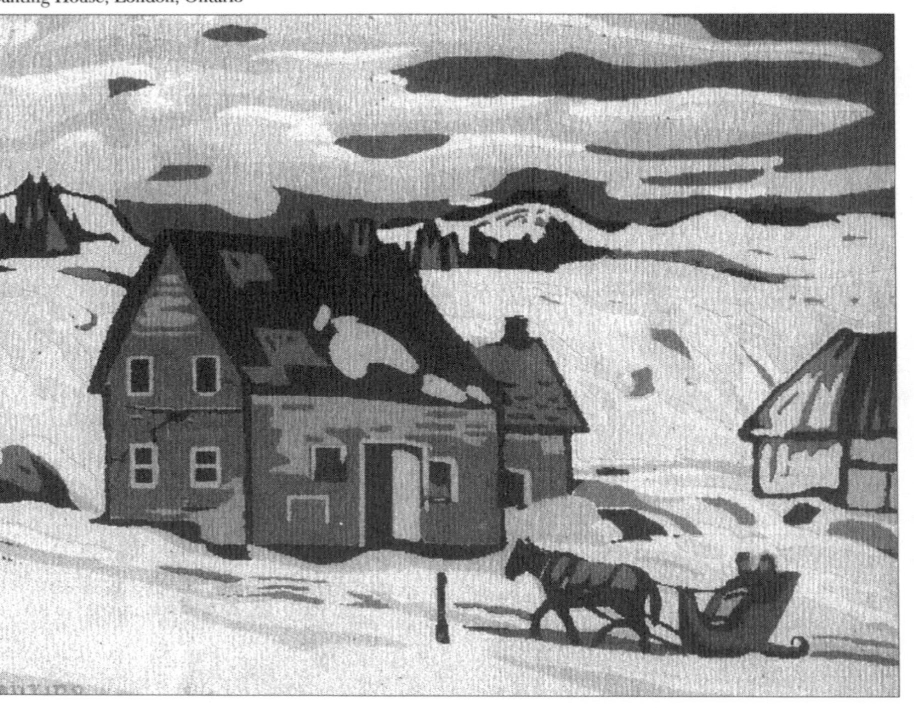

One of Banting's Quebec winter scenes, which he completed
on a painting expedition with Group of Seven artist, A.Y. Jackson.

the spring of 1924 he knew he had nothing to offer. It was not another insulin story.

Anti-vivisectionists were outraged at his experiments and accused him of treating dogs and other animals cruelly. Marion was unhappy, too, but for other reasons. She felt he did not care about her needs. When she was having tea with friends, he'd come in the house smelling of dogs, with dog hair on his clothes. He would refuse to be polite to her guests, and would sit down at the dinner table without changing the suit he had worn in the lab. He did not seem to have anything interesting or witty to say. She wanted to go out in the evening and dance and meet interesting people. He wanted to stay at home and smoke his pipe, have a drink or two. For his part, he disliked her charming friends and thought they were silly and superficial.

Banting turned his attention to cancer research. He had wondered about finding a cure for cancer since 1922. He decided to study Rous sarcoma, a cancerous tumour produced in chickens. It seemed to be caused by a virus. The idea was simple. He would transmit the cancer – named after cancer researcher Peyton Rous – to laboratory chickens. Then he would try to find a vaccine or antitoxin to fight the cancer. If all cancer was like Rous sarcoma, he surmised, and was transmittable, then it could be cured. The work was slow. He used purebred Plymouth Rock chickens and had to order special equipment and microscopes. From 1928 to 1933, tumour-causing material was transplanted into nearly two thousand chickens in Banting's lab. Some of the chickens seemed to resist cancer, but the results were inconclusive.

He needed time to think. He began to spend more time in his third-floor study, smoking his pipe, reading detective stories and painting pictures. The room reeked of oil paints, turpentine, and pipe smoke. For Banting, it was paradise.

From Marion's view, Banting was coarse and did not appreciate the fine things in life. His use of swear words offended her.

One night, while they were dressing for dinner, she said: "We're going to be late. My friends are probably already there."

"I can't tie this bloody tie," he said.

"Here, let me."

"No, I can do it. Damn!"

"You look good in a tuxedo."

"No one ever had a good idea while wearing one of these monkey suits."

"You're a success now, Fred. Start acting like one, and stop behaving like a boy."

"Why don't you start acting like a wife, the way a wife is supposed to act."

Each time they spoke, the distance between them grew a little greater, until finally they were so far apart they couldn't hear what the other person was saying. Banting told his friends the woman he wanted for a wife would be faithful, like an Airedale. But Marion was a "modern" woman, outgoing and opinionated. They fought almost all the time now. She accused him of hitting her. At public functions and dinners the Bantings kept up the appearance of marital happiness. But in their dreamhouse, they slept in separate rooms.

In the Canada of the 1920s, it was difficult for couples to end a bad marriage. Canadians were proud of the fact that they had fewer divorces than Americans, with their tabloid scandals and Hollywood parties. Adultery was considered the only legitimate grounds for divorce, and even a divorce based on adultery was difficult to obtain. Respectable Canadians did not get divorced.

Banting's study had a large library of medical books and books on Canadian history. He was interested in the culture and medicine of Canadian Aboriginal Peoples. He had his briar pipes to smoke and his plain-tipped Buckingham cigarettes and a bottle of whisky that he had stashed away for late-night imbibing when he was writing in his journals. Here, in his study, he could think and create to his heart's content. It was almost like living in the boarding house room during the days back in 1921 when he discovered insulin. He had started drinking diluted laboratory alcohol during that famous struggle, and was still drinking too much. He was also addicted to tobacco, and loved to smoke a pipe, often carving his initials in the bottom of the bowl. He was careful not to advertise his smoking habit. When schoolchildren wrote and asked for a photograph, they would be sent an official picture of a smiling Banting, minus the cigarettes and pipe.

During this period, he wanted to be an author. His favourite reading was not the history of diabetes, but detective fiction. He wanted to be like Arthur Conan Doyle, the physician and creator of Sherlock Holmes. Banting created a fictional sleuth called Silas Eagles, a half-Indian Canadian with an interest in chemistry and all the keen senses of a Holmes. Silas, like Banting, was a lonely man who relaxed by painting. He smoked, worked in a laboratory, and observed people with detachment.

Banting tried to have one of his stories published. It was called, "Si and the Cold Draught." The victim in the story dies by drinking liquid air. The International Magazine Company in 1927 rejected the story as being too reminiscent of Sherlock Holmes. The magazine recommended that Banting find someone who could help him find his way through the dark forest of plot and character development.

Banting had natural talent as a writer. It showed when he wrote about his life and the things he knew. He began to sketch out an autobiography. He wrote about his family, life on their Ontario farm, and the struggle to survive the harsh winters.

He made his first trip to western Canada in 1926, giving a speech to a meeting of the Canadian Medical Association in Victoria, British Columbia. On the trip back, the conductor made an unscheduled stop at a small station in British Columbia.

The passengers on the transcontinental train wondered why they had stopped. They looked out the windows and saw forests and snowcapped mountains. Then a man with a black bag walked off the train. It was Banting. He was met at the station by another physician, who drove him away in a truck. One of the settlers, a diabetic man, was gravely ill, and Banting was there to give a diagnosis and advise the physician on treatment. Banting was in his element. He was happiest when he was healing the sick. It could be on a battlefield with shells falling all around, or in the remote mountains of British Columbia. This was what he was made for, not going to parties or making after-dinner speeches to dignitaries.

ꝏ

Banting had become friends with Group of Seven artist A. Y. Jackson, having met him through the Arts and Letters Club in Toronto, an all-male, exclusive dining and drinking club. In March of 1927, Jackson invited Banting to come with him to Quebec on a sketching trip. The two men painted in the village of St. Jean Port Jolie on the south shore of the St. Lawrence, below Quebec City, in the freezing cold. Banting loved the rugged life. It was the first of many sketching trips the two would take together. Banting always went on these trips under an alias, Frederick Grant, so that he wouldn't be recognized. Grant was his mother's maiden name.

He applied to the Department of the Interior to serve as medical officer aboard the steamer *Beothic*, which was resupplying settlements and RCMP posts in the Eastern Arctic. Banting's friend, A.Y. Jackson, was going on the trip to paint, and Banting wanted to join him.

A week before the steamer sailed, in the summer of 1927, the department sent Banting a telegram: "Can offer nothing luxurious. If you are prepared to face hazards of the north and assume the responsibility Department will be glad to have you." Banting didn't forget Marion. He gave her money for a trip to the British Isles while he was gone.

When Banting's Arctic voyage ended, his marital difficulties were still waiting for him in Toronto. He and Marion tried to work out their problems and set their marriage on a true course. In April, 1929, they had a son, William. But the marriage was beyond repair.

Not long after the baby was born, he told Marion, "I want to live my life the way I want."

She asked him what she was supposed to do now that he wanted to live outside the boundaries of the marriage.

"I suggest you do the same," he said.

Banting began to see a freelance writer in Toronto, Blodwen Davies. She wrote travel literature and met Banting while researching the medical evidence surrounding the mysterious death by drowning of artist Tom Thomson in Algonquin Park, in the woods of northern Ontario. Banting introduced her to Marion and began inviting her to dinner at their house.

Blodwen persuaded Banting to attend meetings of the Toronto Theosophical Society. A few painters, artists, and members of the Arts and Letters Club were members of the society. One of the Theosophist principles was that people can be receptive to mystical insights about the nature of the universe. Theosophy was in vogue, especially among the art crowd and the upper classes. Blodwen told Banting the idea for insulin had come to him as a mystical revelation. She believed that Banting, like the Canadian painters Lawren Harris and Tom Thomson, had achieved a kind of cosmic consciousness. Banting was not a Theosophist, but he yearned to achieve another scientific breakthrough like insulin. He thought and thought, waiting for another great idea. He was a good fisherman, and he compared the process to fishing. Fishermen have to wait for the fish to take the lure. Sometimes they have to wait a long time, but when the strike comes it is worth it.

Silicosis was one area where Banting's post-insulin research was effective. He became the chairman of a research program that produced pioneering studies on the subject. Miners suffered from the disease, a chronic condition marked by fibrosis of the lungs and shortness of breath. Usually fatal, silicosis was brought about by the inhalation of silica particles underground. Banting's name appears on few of the articles produced by the research. He was always careful not to take credit for another researcher's work. In some academic circles, especially in Europe, it was normal for the head of a department to share credit on research. Banting still felt burned by his insulin experience with Macleod. He didn't think that Macleod deserved a share of the Nobel Prize.

In 1931, Fred and Marion were at a party at Blodwen's. Marion was introduced to Donat M. LeBourdais, who worked for the Canadian National Committee on Mental Hygiene. In the months that followed, she met him several times socially and visited him at his nearby Yorkville Avenue apartment to talk about music and art.

LeBourdais had been giving radio broadcasts on mental health for a Toronto radio station, CFRB. In the early evening of Monday, February 8, 1932, Marion visited LeBourdais at his apartment to read the transcript of a broadcast she had missed. They were seated on the couch.

Suddenly, a fist smashed through the glass panel of the apartment door.

Marion jumped off the couch and backed up against the wall. A hand reached in and opened the door from the inside. In rushed Banting and two detectives he had hired from H.A. Sherman Ltd. Secret Service.

"What are you –" But before LeBourdais could get the words out, Banting had him by the throat and was pushing him over the back of the couch to the floor. One of the detectives pulled Banting off the terrified man.

Banting wheeled around and faced Marion, who was still pressed against the wall.

"I want a divorce!" Banting shouted.

Marion nodded, and began to cry.

Banting spent the night with a friend. The next day he picked up his clothes from his home.

Under the absurd laws of the time, it was often necessary to prove immoral or adulterous behaviour before legal proceedings for a divorce could go ahead. That explains, in part, Banting's decision to hire private detectives.

On February 10, two days later, a notice appeared in the classified ads of the *Toronto Star*. The notice said that F.G. Banting, M.D., formerly of 46 Bedford Road, Toronto, would not be responsible for any debts made in his name, after that date, without his written order.

A divorce was sure to ruin Banting's position at the university and his standing in the medical profession. A divorce would also damage Marion's social position and reputation.

The lawyers for both sides met. The Bantings were assured there would be no publicity. Marion decided not to defend herself against Banting's divorce action. He would give her $250 a month, custody of their son Bill, and possession of the house. On April 25, a judge quietly granted them a decree which stipulated that their divorce would become final in six months. But the year before, in 1931, divorce actions had been transferred from federal jurisdiction to the Supreme Court of Ontario. Under the new law, the press had more freedom to report on divorce actions. The Toronto *Telegram* published a front-page account of the divorce proceedings, describing the raid on LeBourdais' apartment. The story was out. Now that the *Telegram* had published an account, the *Star* and other newspapers would have to follow. That was how newspapers worked. They didn't have a personal vendetta against Banting. He was news, juicy news. His divorce was like one of those Hollywood scandals that Canadians were always wagging their fingers at.

In October, one week before the divorce was to become final, LeBourdais and William Robertson, Marion's father, filed motions of intervention. Robertson believed Banting had been having an affair, and that he had been physically abusive to Marion during their marriage. He did not want his daughter's reputation ruined. LeBourdais denied the detectives' testimony that they had entered a darkened apartment and flashed a light around.

In November, the front page headline of the *Telegram*'s evening edition said: "Dr. Banting Cruel to Wife, Father Claims." The *Star* newspaper wanted to match the story and sent a reporter to interview Banting, but the Nobel laureate refused to talk.

A judge heard the motions of intervention from Marion's father and LeBourdais. But the divorce went ahead as planned and was granted in December, 1932.

Fred had wanted to be a respected family man just like his father. Now he was accused in the press of being an adulterer and wife beater. Marion kept the name Banting and continued to live at Bedford Road. Then she moved to Oakville, outside of Toronto, and went back to work, becoming the head of the shoppers' service at Simpson's Department Store. Their son Bill visited Fred on weekends.

Despite his divorce and the scandal in the newspapers, Banting continued to be showered with awards, honours, medals, and memberships.

The Conservative Prime Minister of Canada, R.B. Bennett, renewed the granting of titles to Canadians, a practice which had been suspended in 1919. In the King's birthday honours list, released in June, 1934, the title of Knight Commander of the Civil Division of the Order of the British Empire was given to Dr. Fred Banting, the hero of insulin. He was now Sir Frederick Banting, K.B.E. The knighthood made Banting uncomfortable. However, it showed that he had not been disgraced by divorce.

Banting told friends that anyone who called him "Sir Frederick" would get a kick in the ass.

He now lived quietly in an apartment near the university, with a housekeeper to cook and clean.

For the rest of his life, Banting continued to work on research projects but only found peace of mind in rural Canada, far from civilization. He enjoyed tramping around in the cold and finding a scene to paint, a barn, a tree, a rectangle of window light falling on snow. He painted on birch panels until his fingers froze. The villages and farms in Quebec reminded him of his boyhood farm in Ontario.

Although he worked on scientific research, Banting disliked the modern world. He grew up with the Methodist ethic and its emphasis on hard work. He was contemptuous of upper-class society. He no longer believed in organized religion, but was the product of his hard-working parents and books like *The Pilgrim's Progress*. Christian, the hero of that book, has to navigate his own Vanity Fair, and makes it clear that success is bought at the price of suffering and inner conflict. Laziness and despair were his enemies. Undesirable characters in *The Pilgrim's Progress* were always members of the aristocracy or landed gentry. The Pilgrim was a labouring man.

Banting was not considered a brilliant researcher. He sometimes made comparisons between medical research and detective work and believed researchers should be like Sherlock Holmes, or "secret service" men. Science, for Banting, existed in the world of intuition, hard work, and sweat. He thought scientists should have keen powers of observation and be informed of everything on the subjects they planned to investigate. Ironically, when he discovered insulin, he might have had keen powers of observation, but he had almost no working knowledge of the subject.

His didn't believe in the God of his parents, but he sometimes believed the Creator could be seen and experienced in Nature. His moral code, though strict, was based on a double standard when it came to Marion, his wife. He worried what his mother would think of the divorce, and was relieved when she said it was for the best.

He had survived. He had come through his divorce with barely a scratch, except for the newspapers that had dragged his personal life through the muck. He would never understand, or forgive, the press. Let the press be hanged. He was on top of the world. But if he thought his troubles lay behind him, he was mistaken. The discovery of insulin, and the fame it brought, had set the stage for years of turmoil.

7

The Great Utopia and the Ministry of Love

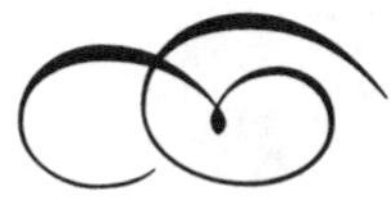

In October, 1929, the New York Stock Exchange collapsed. Banks shut their doors, and ordinary citizens lost their life savings. Factories went idle, and prices for food crops plummeted. Farmers could not repay their bank loans and were forced off their land. A full-scale economic depression spread across the United States, Canada, Europe, and the rest of the world. The Great Depression continued through the 1930s, affecting daily life everywhere.

At one time, Banting, like other idealists in North America, believed the Depression was a clear sign that the capitalist economic system did not work. Some

10102. TR-2000-41. Courtesy of Simcoe County Archives & New Tecumseth Public Library.

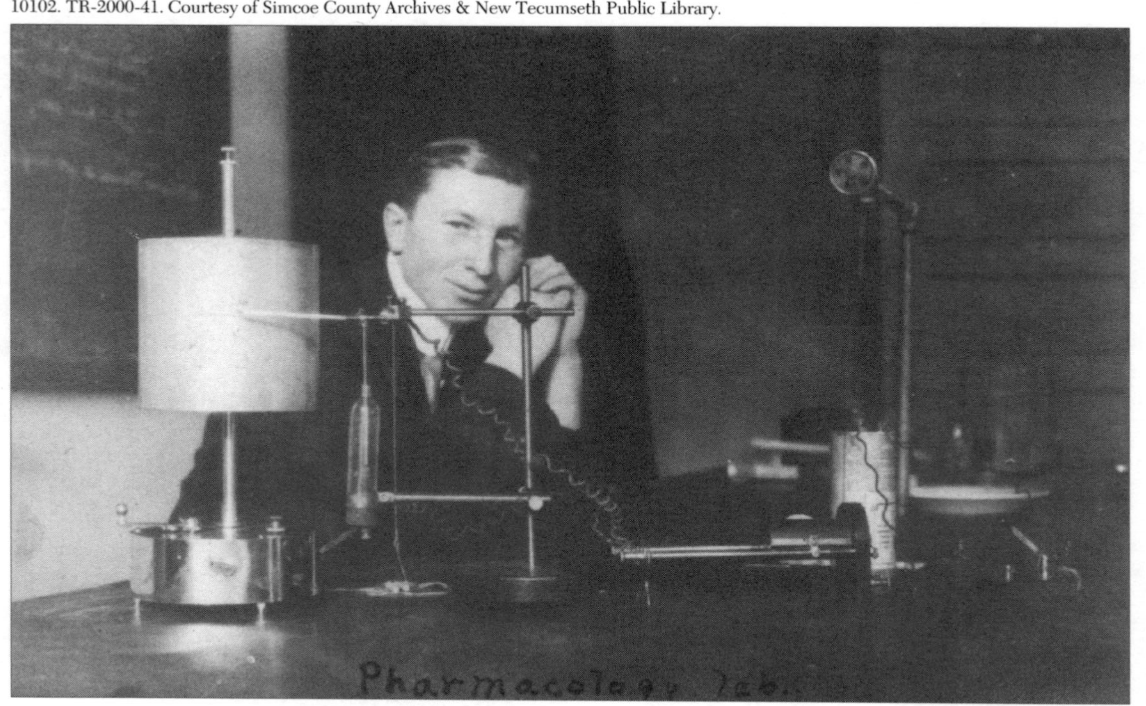

A confident Banting at ease in his laboratory.

people looked to the Soviet Union, believing it could solve the world's problems.

The Soviet Union boasted that the 1917 Bolshevik revolution had transformed society into a socialist utopia, an ideal world where hunger and crime did not exist. Banting was fascinated by these developments. In some respects, he thought the democratic system in Canada and the United States was a farce. He liked the way the Soviets controlled their newspapers. He had nothing good to say about a free press. During his divorce, the press had kicked him when he was down.

In the 1930s, Banting wanted to repeat his insulin success in the laboratory. He also tried to sort out his troubled life. He broke off his relationship with Blodwen, who fled, broken, from Toronto. She had criticized his anger and his grudges. She felt his negative emotions were blocking access to higher, more creative thinking, and accused him of fumbling around in the dark. But that was fine with him. He didn't like fancy parties, and he especially didn't like airy intellectuals. He may have had his idea for insulin in the middle of the night, but he didn't believe all that Theosophy stuff.

He took a short sketching trip to Cape Cod, along the Massachusetts coast. He visited the Deaconess Hospital in Boston where Dr. Elliott Joslin had his diabetic practice. There he met Joslin's associate, Dr. Priscilla White. They met for the second time at a medical conference in Montreal and went sleigh-riding. But they eventually drifted apart.

Banting left Canada in 1933 for a two-month European trip. He attended the International Cancer

Congress in Madrid, but disliked the academic social climbing he saw at the meeting. He thought about his research, went to a bullfight, and used his spare time to sketch the trees and the old buildings. He thought it was a fine country to paint. He waited for more brilliant ideas. He believed if he waited long enough, he would have another one. He was like a fisherman, but he was fishing for ideas. He believed he should be always ready for the strike at the end of the fishing line.

In 1935, he sailed across the Atlantic to be inducted into the prestigious Royal Society of London. Then he planned to go from England to Russia, where he would attend the Fifteenth Physiological Congress in Leningrad. He wanted to see this great utopia everyone was talking about.

On June 22, he left London for Leningrad aboard the U.S.S.R. steamship *Smolny*, which was decorated with red carpets, red tablecloths, and portraits of Marx, Engels, Lenin, and Stalin.

Banting was not aware that the country's ruler, Stalin, was terrorizing Russian citizens. He believed that Russia supported art and artists. He did not know that artists were often the first victims of the socialist crackdown. As the steamship sailed on, he tried to keep an open mind and dutifully listened to lectures on Russian political achievement. He couldn't help but be impressed with a country that boasted no unemployment in the 1930s, when in Toronto there were people without jobs who had to wait in long soup lines for something to eat.

In Russia, Banting and his travelling companions were accompanied by official tourist guides everywhere they went. Banting paid a visit to the country's greatest scientist, I.P. Pavlov, the physiologist and behaviorist. Pavlov was eighty-five years old. His health had not been good. After touring Pavlov's Institute of Experimental Medicine, Banting and his companions were driven to the old man's villa outside Leningrad.

Uniformed guards came out to meet the car and open the huge iron gates.

Banting stepped out of the car into the courtyard and looked around. Suddenly, there was an enormous crash. Nearby was a large iron cage containing two enormous gorillas. The male gorilla was upset at the arrival of the strangers, and was shaking the cage as if he meant to break it apart. A boy came with a whip, and the gorilla quieted down.

Banting and the others were ushered upstairs, and Pavlov rushed forward to meet them. The old man, his white beard jumping up and down as he laughed, led them down a hall to his study, where he sat on a couch and complained to Banting about his various health problems.

Banting had pictured Pavlov as a quiet, pensive man. Instead, the old fellow was garrulous and animated. Banting felt sorry for him. In his old age he had become a cultural icon, imprisoned in his palace like a gorilla in a cage for all to see.

Banting got back to his room at the Hotel National just in time to see a parade of singing athletes in the street below. For two hours, they marched and sang, carrying rifles and huge pictures of Lenin and Stalin. Warplanes roared over the hotel. Banting was impressed.

Banting wasn't the only Canadian at the Physiological Congress, which opened August 8. Dr. Norman Bethune, one of Banting's medical school classmates, was there. Bethune and Banting were almost the same age. They had been born about 250 kilometres apart in rural Ontario, north of Toronto. They had both been wounded in war, had become surgeons, and were divorced. Like Banting, Bethune had abandoned organized Christianity. They both liked to paint, but where Banting's pictures were pastoral, Bethune's were angry and dark. There was another difference. In 1935, Banting was famous and Bethune was just a surgeon from Montreal. Bethune had not yet come to believe in Communism as a kind of religion, nor had he gone to China. He would achieve fame as a surgeon to Communist Chinese guerrilla forces fighting Japanese invaders, and in 1939 he would die of blood poisoning in China.

Banting spent most of July 1935 touring the Soviet Union by rail and boat. The tourist guides were careful to showcase only the best apartment buildings and factories. Banting noticed poor housing and shoddy huts and children with protruding abdomens, a sign of starvation. He observed that waiting rooms in some railway stations were beautifully furnished for officials and "first-class foreigners," despite the Soviet claim that class distinctions did not exist. On a boat trip across the Black Sea, only first- and second-class passengers had sleeping berths, and the toilets on the boat, he noticed, were filthy.

He couldn't wait to get home. When he tried to board the *Siberia*, sailing from Leningrad to London, he was told there was no room. Tourist officials promised to send him home by plane, but bad weather made flying out of the question. Finally, he was put on a slow train heading west. The train crossed through Poland and through Germany, where he saw swastika flags flying everywhere over the neat, clean fields.

At the end of August, 1935, he arrived back in London. Four days later he left for Canada. In another five years, the countryside he had just visited would be overrun with war, soldiers, and refugees.

Banting admired the Soviet system of socialized medicine. When he compared science in the Soviet Union with the treatment of research in his native country, the U.S.S.R. came out on top. The way he saw it, Canada was controlled by the newspapers and the rich. Public opinion was everything. The creators who worked in science and the arts had to beg the government for money, yet had no voice in the way the country was run.

He began calling himself a communist and referring to his friends as "comrade." His friends soon grew tired of it. After giving a few interviews to the newspapers about the benefits of Soviet society, he stopped praising the U.S.S.R.

Banting never joined the Communist party. He was not a communist, a theosophist, or a methodist. He was a man of simple tastes who happened to do one great thing that changed people's lives forever.

Banting believed that Russian totalitarian society crushed the individual. If he had lived long enough to see the publication of George Orwell's *1984*, he probably would have understood the predicament of Winston, the novel's hero, who works at the Ministry of Truth. The Ministry of Truth was responsible for spreading lies and propaganda. The Ministry of Love was a building with no windows. The worst crimes were to think, and to love.

8

Painting Till His Fingers Froze

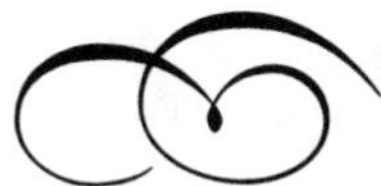

Banting couldn't sleep. He was in his study, painting a picture of a winter scene in Quebec. A horse was pulling a sleigh. He painted the sleigh red. He had to laugh. He suddenly remembered the time when he was in Toronto, working on insulin, and had painted more snow onto a picture of maple sugaring that hung in the hallway of his boarding house. Banting believed that scientists, like certain painters, were artists. He saw himself as an artist. He believed that scientists were creators, and that they shared with artists a kind of renegade psychology that put them on the fringes of society.

In the early 1920s a Canadian art movement was making waves in Toronto. The Group of Seven, friends

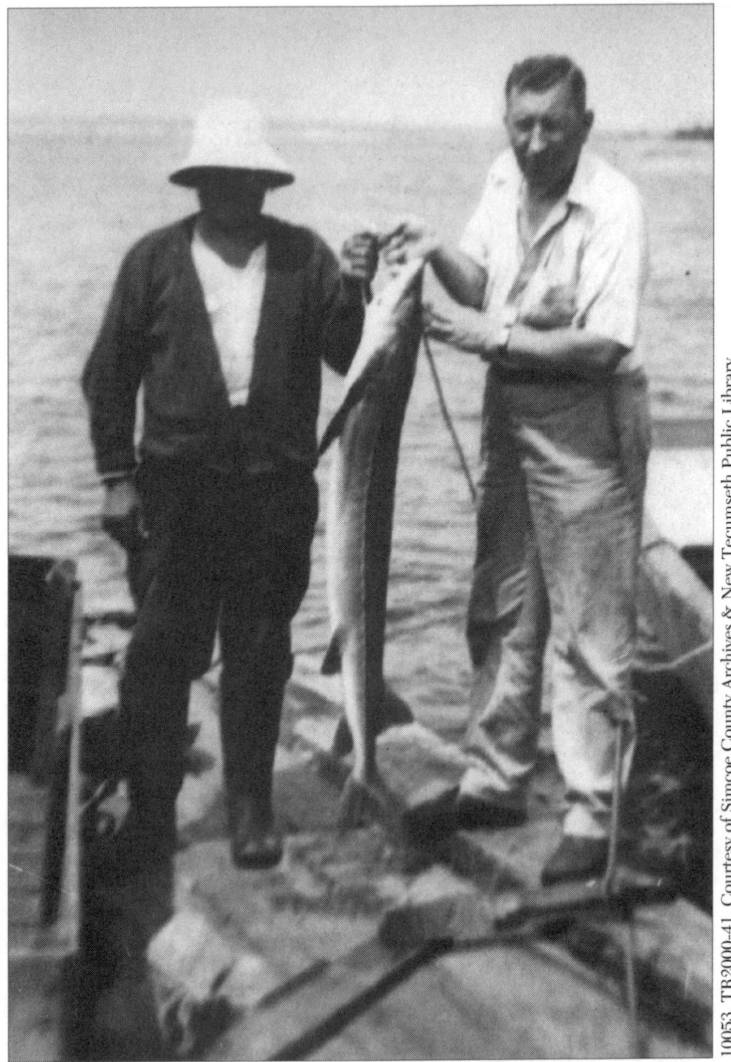

10053. TR2000-41. Courtesy of Simcoe County Archives & New Tecumseth Public Library.

Banting, the complete angler – but ideas in his later years were harder to catch than fish.

of Tom Thomson, an artist who had painted in Algonquin Park and drowned in the park's Canoe Lake, set out deliberately to upset the conventions of Canadian art. The artists saw themselves as rebels. Banting identified with this image of the outsider who has to fight society to make his views known. Didn't he fight Macleod and the other bureaucrats in Toronto every step of the way just to bring insulin to the world? And didn't he have to go to New York to get money to buy equipment to make insulin, when Toronto turned him down? Even his original idea to develop an extract for diabetics received a cold shoulder at first from people like Macleod, who was part of the establishment.

In January, 1925, two years after he won the Nobel Prize and was financially secure, Banting contributed two small canvases to an exhibit of the work of University of Toronto staff and students. The *Star Weekly* saw the influence of the Group of Seven in his paintings. But it also said the only school Banting seemed to represent was the "Medical School."

Around this time, Banting met Lawren Harris, a Group of Seven artist. In April of 1925 Harris nominated Banting for membership in the Arts and Letters Club of Toronto, which was located within walking distance of the university.

Members of the social and dining club included the Group of Seven and many of the group's admirers and critics. Women were not permitted to be members. Banting liked the singing, skits, and fellowship of drinking men. In some ways, it reminded him of the camaraderie he experienced during the war.

The greatest friend of Banting's life was the painter A.Y. Jackson, whom he met through the Arts and Letters Club. Jackson was a lifelong bachelor, eight years older than Banting.

In 1927, when Banting and Jackson travelled aboard the *Beothic* to resupply RCMP posts in the Arctic, they shared a stateroom with a government botanist, O.M. Malte. Malte had brought along a supply of rum which he had purchased from bootleggers before leaving port in North Sydney, Nova Scotia.

From the deck of the ship, painting in oils on small wooden panels, Banting and Jackson tried to capture icebergs, waves, shadows, and the play of light on ice and snow.

The *Beothic* steamed north through the Davis Strait and Baffin Bay, dropping off supplies at the most northern outpost in the world, the RCMP station on the Bache Peninsula of Ellesmere Island. Bad weather socked them in at Beechey Island, where Sir John Franklin and his men spent their last winter in 1845-46.

The ship sailed on with Malte in the ship's saloon, poring over specimens with a magnifying glass, and celebrating with a drink each time he discovered a new variety of moss or fern, or a plant that grew in the far north, where it shouldn't exist.

"Malte! Look what we found!" Jackson shouted.

The botanist looked up from his table as Jackson and Banting trudged into the saloon. They had been exploring on one of the islands, and had found another plant for the botanist.

"What do you think?" asked Banting. "Is it a good one?"

"My goodness," Malte said, staring at the leafy herb. "Let me see."

They handed him the plant.

"Ha!"

"I suppose that means it's suitable," Banting said.

"Quite rare," said Malte.

"It's a beauty all right," Jackson said.

"This calls for a celebration," Malte said, gingerly making his way back to the table strewn with plants and papers.

"Not another celebration," Jackson said, grinning.

"Another round," Banting said. "In the name of botany."

Banting listened carefully as the men on board the *Beothic* talked about Canada's expeditions, the shoddy supplies dropped off at police posts, and the fate of the Inuit in the white man's Arctic. Once upon a time, the Inuit had followed the caribou in their migrations. Now the Aboriginal People had become dependent on Hudson's Bay Company stores for many of their needs. Some of the Mounties told him that the Hudson's Bay Company fur traders were only interested in how much money they could make from the Inuit. Banting compared the makeshift clothing of the Inuit with the beautiful furs the company bought in trade for tea and tobacco. He thought that some of the profit that was being made on furs should be given to the Inuit. Much of their food was canned, obtained by barter in company stores. Banting believed white man's food was not good for the Inuit.

As the *Beothic* steamed south through the Labrador Sea, six weeks after the voyage began,

Banting looked out at the ice floes and thought about the treatment of the Inuit. The Arctic didn't seem beautiful anymore. He and Jackson stopped sketching.

The *Toronto Star*'s Roy Greenaway, the paper's hotshot reporter who broke the story of insulin, met Banting in Montreal. The two men took the train back to Toronto. Greenaway interviewed Banting on the train and wrote a short piece about the Arctic trip. Banting had promised not to talk to the press without clearing it first with the Department of the Interior. He looked over Greenaway's piece and decided it was fine.

When the train stopped at Kingston, Greenaway wired his material to Toronto. But when he got back on the train, Banting opened up and told him what he really thought about the Hudson's Bay Company, and how the Aboriginal People in the north were being exploited. Greenaway could smell a good story a mile away. He was taking notes, and thought Banting knew his comments were on the record.

The next day the headline in the *Toronto Star* read: "Banting Regrets Hudson Bay Use Of Eskimo." The story contained Banting's charges, and his comment that there was barely one real Canadian among the foreigners in the Hudson's Bay Company. The most famous person in Canada had just fired a broadside at one of the country's most established and prestigious businesses.

The Governors of the Hudson's Bay Company called the charges slanderous. The company said Banting was naive to believe that the Inuit were simple, healthy children of nature who would have been better off had they never come into contact with civilization.

The Department of the Interior told the press that Banting's views were in poor taste because he was a guest and had promised not to make any comments to the press without the department's approval. Banting was furious with Greenaway. He felt the press had kicked him again.

Banting eventually submitted two reports to the Department of the Interior on the health of the Inuit. He did not change the story he told Greenaway. He said white man's food was bad for the Inuit diet, white man's clothing was useless in the bitter climate, and fur trading would someday lead to the extinction of the Inuit.

In 1928, with his marriage faltering, and nothing dramatic happening with his lab work, Banting went with Jackson to explore and sketch on the Great Slave Lake. Droves of mosquitoes and blackflies pursued them and landed in their paint. Canada's Nobel laureate couldn't even find peace in the woods.

Back in Toronto, J.J.R. Macleod, the professor of physiology who had guided Banting's insulin team, decided to return to Scotland. He had shared the Nobel Prize with Banting, but Banting's refusal to acknowledge his contribution – Banting shared his half of the prize with Best, and considered turning down the award altogether because Macleod had been named the co-winner – continued to haunt him.

To his friends, Macleod communicated his bitterness. He was a hero in Scotland, and was offered the Regius Chair in Physiology at his home university in Aberdeen. Macleod had had a brilliant career as a researcher, but he was fed up with Canada, especially Banting and the bureaucracy at the University of

Toronto. Macleod and Banting never worked together on another project again. All they ever shared after the Nobel Prize was a wall of paintings at the university's Hart House, during an exhibition of amateur art. Banting did not attend Macleod's farewell dinner before he left for Scotland. Macleod never set foot in Canada again. He died in 1935.

As for Best, the thirty-two-year-old researcher was made Professor of Physiology in 1929, replacing Macleod. Over the years, Banting grew to dislike Best. He felt the young researcher had become a slave to ambition in the highly charged academic and research world of the University of Toronto. After a productive research career, Best retired in 1967 and died eleven years later.

Collip, a brilliant chemist, studied hormones and became one of Canada's leading endocrinologists. He said publicly that his contribution to the insulin research was small, but as the years passed, Banting always told people that the research couldn't have been done without him. Collip died in 1965 at age seventy-two.

Back in 1921, when Best was Banting's student assistant on the diabetes project, he lived with his aunt in Toronto. She wrote Banting an angry letter in 1923 asking if he was responsible for spreading the report that it was Banting "and" Best, not Banting "with" Best, who had discovered insulin. She wanted to know why Banting's part in the discovery was so much more valuable than her nephew's.

Wearily, and with considerable tact, he replied that Best's name was sometimes not mentioned with his because he sometimes had to lecture and present papers on the clinical aspect of the research, and that newspapers had, at times, used their names separately.

Collip's supporters in Alberta, in the Canadian west, believed the Eastern media had ignored his contributions. But the idea that started it all, and the passion that motivated it, was Banting's.

Banting made sure in the beginning that people knew insulin was his idea. But he did not have to spend a lot of time fostering his worldwide reputation. The glory and fame for discovering insulin followed him like a shadow. Not only was he the most famous person in Canada, he was famous throughout the world. Everyone wanted to meet him, from poor people to kings. It was assumed that he was an expert on diabetes, but others, like the American diabetologist Elliott Joslin, were the experts. Even Mackenzie King, the Canadian prime minister, referred diabetic friends to Banting.

Banting had a complex relationship with fame. He nurtured it, but it disgusted him. Fame was a two-edged sword, and Banting had to be careful how he used the blade, or it would cut him. He wanted to leave insulin behind, but couldn't. He was only happy when he was painting outdoors, perhaps in the snow, or cooking his food over a campfire, or smoking his pipe beneath the stars in a remote village in Quebec. Then he felt free.

Years later, the painter A.Y. Jackson wrote a little book, *Banting As An Artist*, in which he reminisced about some of their sketching trips. Of the *Beothic* journey, he wrote: *We accumulated a lot of material. Studies of icebergs, glaciers, floe-ice and the rugged coastline, and more intimate stuff when we got ashore. Sometimes we would find ourselves working at one or two o'clock in the morning. The twenty-four hours of daylight was demoralizing. As we went south there seemed to be more variety to the light and the cloud forms and it was good to have night again. Banting's sketches on the trip, the longest time he had ever spent sketching, showed a lot of promise. I would josh him about dropping science and turning to art. "When I am fifty, that's what I intend to do," he would say. He believed researching was a job for young men, and that his duty was to create favourable conditions for them to work under. In 1930 we went to Saint-Fidèle, a little village below Murray Bay. Across the wide river we could see the low hills of the south shore and the great fields of ice drifting up or down, with the tides. It was an humble little village and the fare was simple but wholesome and generous. There were detective stories to read in the long evenings. There was almost daily correspondence with the "lab" regarding a hen which was immune to cancer. He sketched continually in all sorts of weather and was pleased with a word of approval. But his usual question, when he showed me a sketch, was "Now what's wrong with it?" There were long hikes on the roads or across country on snowshoes, lunch with a fire on top of the snow to warm ourselves and toast our sandwiches, and tea made in a lard pail.*

When they made their sketching trips to the Quebec countryside they had no responsibilities, except to observe and paint. They dressed in old wool clothes and cooked their meals outdoors, in the bitter cold, over campfires. Banting would sooner or later run out of Buckingham cigarettes and start smoking one of the French-Canadian brands. He liked the "atmosphere" of Rose Quesnel cigarettes, and felt these native smokes helped him express the country better in his paintings. For Banting, smoking pipes or cigarettes was almost an art, a serious form of relaxation, as it was with Sherlock Holmes, his favourite fictional detective.

The sketching trips reminded Banting of the pastoral countryside of his youth. Rural Quebec with its farmhouses and churches was a land forgotten by time, and Banting didn't want to leave. Against this backdrop he looked at his life in Toronto with its endless parties, academic social-climbing, and fancy-dressed men, and despised what he saw.

In Saint-Fidèle, there were no streetlights, and the nights were black. One night Banting and Jackson went for a walk in a driving blizzard. Light shone on the snow from the windows of the houses, but beyond the squares of light there was only darkness. It had been snowing all day, and Banting could not see the drifts. Before he knew it, he was wading thigh-deep in snow. He was reminded of the winters in Ontario when he was a boy.

They took off their gloves and rubbed their hands in front of the fireplace when they got back to the old farmhouse where they were staying.

They talked about the houses they saw on their walk, and the best way to paint them. The fire crackled.

"At least the house is warm," Jackson said.

"It's warm, but it creaks like an old barn in the wind," Banting replied. He lit a Rose Quesnel.

"Let's have a drink before we turn in."

"Good idea," Banting said.

They took turns swigging whisky from a bottle.

"I don't want to leave this country," Banting said.

"The people are good. They work hard. They are not in a hurry," Jackson said.

"But we will have to go back. We will have to go back to civilization."

"It is too bad," Jackson said.

"I swear I am going to come back here someday."

"Perhaps, someday," Jackson said.

"Someday would be good." Banting handed Jackson the bottle. In the glow of the fireplace they drank. Banting lit another cigarette.

On his fortieth birthday, in November, 1931, Banting looked back on his sketching trips. He had sketched in Quebec and the Canadian Rockies. He had painted at Georgian Bay, Baffin Bay, and French River. He had painted at Lake Louise, and at Fort Resolution, N.W.T. He had painted in the Arctic, on the streets of Spain and southern France, and at Gloucester Harbor in Massachusetts. But nothing was the same for Banting as painting in Canada. He felt as if his native country were more precious to him than life. He loved the land, the rivers, mountains and animals. He thought the people who lived in Canada were the best in the world. But he sometimes thought he would prefer his country if there were no people at all.

By the 1930s, Banting had become one of Canada's best known amateur painters. He kept his paintings or gave them away to friends and relatives. His paintings of Quebec barns and snow and trees tended to resemble Jackson's work, with the same strong use of colour and composition. But he also made pen-and-ink drawings when he was in Russia, and cartoon caricatures of his friends, and wood carvings: chests, humidors, and pipe racks. He was laughed at when he tried to sell some of his sketches back in 1920, when he was a struggling doctor. Later, though, some of his paintings appeared in a Canadian Artists Series of Christmas cards published by Rous and Mann. The $13.77 he received in royalties was the only money he ever made from his paintings.

Banting made one more sketching trip with Jackson, to Saint-Tite-des-Cap in March, 1937. But his mind was on his laboratory work, and the political crisis overseas.

War was building in Europe and Asia. Japan invaded China, and a Nazi named Adolf Hitler was preaching hate and winning the admiration of the German people.

Banting wanted to defeat the Nazis. He threw himself into military research and top-secret projects on bacterial warfare. But he would never again sketch in his beloved Quebec.

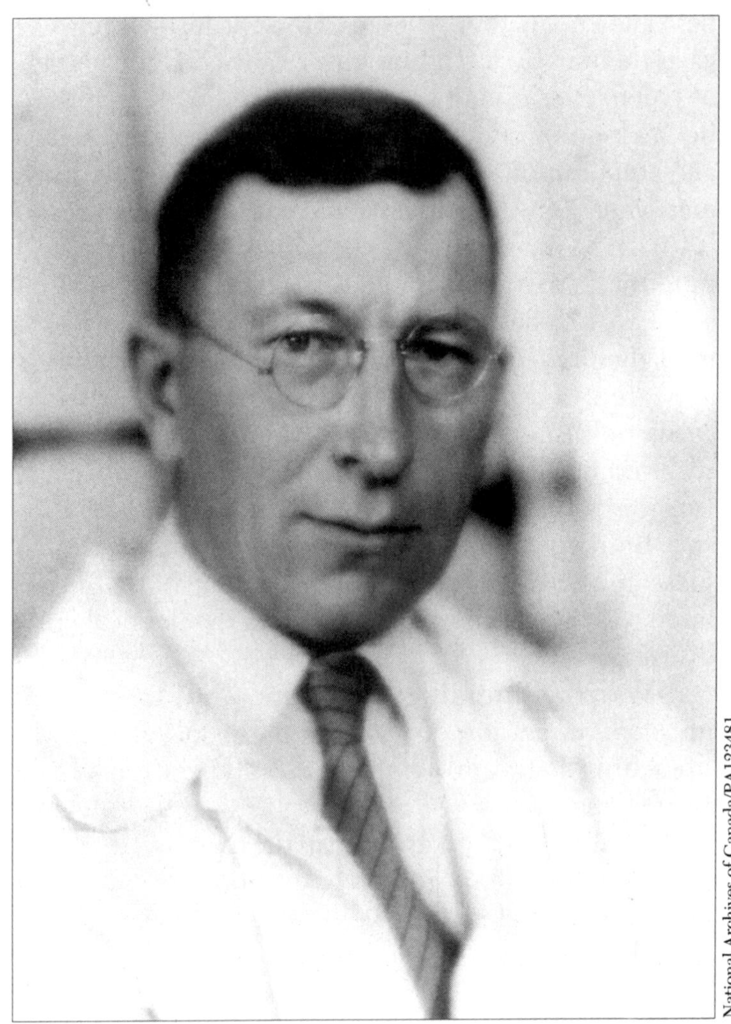

National Archives of Canada/PA123481.

With the onset of the Second World War, and the demands of his fame, Banting found it more and more difficult to work in his lab.

9

Fighting Like a Man

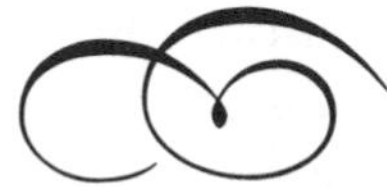

Even before the Second World War began in 1939, Banting had begun to investigate the potential for using bacterial warfare against an enemy. He was worried about Hitler's military buildup in Germany, and he felt that bacterial warfare might be the only way to stop the Nazis.

He had begun to serve on Canada's National Research Council (NRC), a government-funded body that had been formed to co-ordinate scientific research in the country. The head of the NRC was General Andrew McNaughton, who had been a brigadier-general in the First World War. Banting and McNaughton hit it off. They had fought the Germans in World War One. They did not underestimate the enemy. They believed that Hitler wanted to conquer the world.

As a medical researcher and veteran, Banting had been interested for years in the possibility of contaminating an enemy with disease. Poison gas had been used in the First World War, and there were rumours that germ warfare was also used.

Before the war, with Hitler's power growing, McNaughton, the head of the NRC, asked Banting to prepare a memorandum on the subject of bacterial warfare.

Banting's confidential memo, dated September 16, 1937, said it was possible for airplanes to drop waterborne diseases such as typhoid into city reservoirs, and that insect-borne diseases, such as plague, could be spread to enemy troops or civilians. He proposed that deadly viruses could be carried to the enemy by dust bombs.

In the fall of 1938, Banting, as chairman of the NRC's Associate Committee on Medical Research, toured Canada to see what the universities and public health laboratories were doing in the way of scientific research. Banting pleaded for more government money so that young scientists would stay in Canada and not emigrate to the United States, where the prospects for research were brighter.

By 1939, Banting was being pulled a hundred different ways by the demands of his fame, not to mention his work for the NRC. He barely had time for lab work. He had piles of letters to answer, not just from fans who wanted his autograph, but from strangers who wanted money. Reporters wanted exclusive interviews, and anti-vivisectionists wanted Banting's skin.

He was not looking after his own health. He smoked several packs of cigarettes a day. He smoked a pipe, too, and had a chronic cough. He did not believe in exercise, and he had insomnia. He drank alcohol heavily at night to help himself sleep.

In 1936, Banting had moved to a house he bought at 205 Rosedale Heights Drive, overlooking the city of Toronto. He grew roses and liked working in his garden. His son Bill would visit him and he would make up bedtime stories and sometimes he would take the boy to the lab and show him how to decapitate mice.

He was in his late forties now, and his scandalous divorce was behind him. He had much on his mind: his research, his duties on the NRC, and all the minute, boring chores that being famous entailed. He liked drinking with his pals and singing war songs and reminiscing about his friends who had given their lives in the Great War. But he wanted to marry again. He had his eye out for the right woman and was about to embark on another whirlwind romance.

Henrietta Ball, a native of Stanstead, Quebec, had studied science at Mount Allison University in New Brunswick. She had worked for three years in a tuberculosis laboratory in Saint John. She came to the University of Toronto in the 1936-37 academic year and did her work for an MA in the Department of Medical Research.

In 1937, when she was twenty-five and Banting was forty-six, they began to see each other. In the course of their tumultuous relationship, she went to

England to continue her studies. Banting followed her overseas.

They were married in June, 1939. Banting had been knighted for his insulin work, and now he and his wife were known as Sir Frederick and Henrietta, Lady Banting. They spent a short honeymoon on the shores of Georgian Bay before returning to live at Banting's house.

At one time, before the war, Banting had considered researching the health-giving properties of royal jelly, a nutritious secretion of the honeybee that is fed to the very young larvae in a colony and to all queen larvae. He wanted to understand it and see if it could be applied to humans in a beneficial way. But times had changed. He now felt he had to focus on the military use of deadly bacteria and diabolical chemicals.

Then, on September 1, 1939, Hitler invaded Poland. Banting saw that war with Germany was imminent and re-enlisted in the army, signing up as a pathologist with his old unit in the Royal Canadian Medical Corps. Days later, the British Empire was at war with Germany.

During the next six years the Second World War would see the barbaric extermination of six million Jews and other minorities, the fire-bombing of entire cities, and the use of the atom bomb.

In the beginning the Germans used swift, motorized advances, aided by artillery and fighter planes, which they called "blitzkrieg," or "lightning war." In less than a year Hitler's armies had occupied France, Denmark, Norway, Belgium, the Netherlands, and Luxembourg. Greece and Yugoslavia were next to fall.

British troops were driven off the European mainland. Every time Banting heard the news on the radio or read the newspapers, he grew more impatient to fight. The Allies were in a desperate situation.

Banting had re-enlisted so he could be where the fighting was. But his other work was too valuable. He was promoted to major and ordered to continue his military research with the National Research Council.

In England he visited the Ministry of Supply's Chemical Defence Experimental Station at Porton, where the British conducted experiments in gas warfare and antidotes. Banting concluded that the antidote ointment developed there was superior to anything Canada had and cabled the National Research Council in Ottawa to send scientists to Porton rather than trying to duplicate the work.

He was worried that the Germans might try to infect Allied populations with bacteria, either by dropping the material from planes, or by infecting water supplies. He argued that the Allies should take the offensive and use bacterial warfare against the Germans. He was all for developing deterrents, but he thought the enemy should be disabled first. He had several ideas for spreading disease. One of these ideas was to distribute infected propaganda leaflets to the enemy. Another idea was to spread bacteria-laden silica particles among the enemy, creating artificial, but deadly, insect bites.

He proposed that an organization be established to protect people and animals against bacteriological warfare, perhaps with Canada taking the lead role.

Canada's High Commissioner to Great Britain, Vincent Massey, was interested in Banting's ideas.

(Massey's brother, Raymond, was an actor. Among other roles, he would play a patriotic Canadian in the *The 49th Parallel*, a famous 1941 war movie directed by Michael Powell.) Vincent Massey was a friend of Banting's and a fellow member of the Arts and Letters Club in Toronto. He arranged for Banting to see the British minister responsible for chemical and biological warfare. Banting's meeting went well, and he waited in London for an answer. While he waited he went to theatres and watched newsreels and cartoons. At one of these newsreel theatres he saw a film about the discovery of insulin. He hated the film so much he decided to write down his own story. He wrote about 30,000 words in longhand just to set the record straight.

He eventually learned that his proposal for a bacteriological warfare research centre did not have the support of British bureaucrats and research scientists. They did not believe the Germans would ever use germ warfare. If they did, the bureaucrats said, it wouldn't work.

Banting sailed for home at the end of January, 1940. The ship's departure was announced on the radio by Lord Haw Haw, the German propagandist, as its last voyage. But the only problem the passengers encountered was seasickness. As he sailed home, Banting thought his proposal for a research centre had failed for good. No one in Britain or Canada seemed to know what to do with it. He did not know that the British continued to discuss his ideas. A year later, in 1941, a microbiological research station was established at Porton.

ꟹ

In June, 1940, Banting began to explore different ways to spread biological agents among an enemy. In July, the Minister of National Defence approved Banting's proposal to investigate this issue. He met with a group of bacteriologists and virologists at the University of Toronto, including experts from Connaught Laboratories, which had helped Banting mass-produce insulin.

The group talked about the best types of material for carrying bacteria or viruses into enemy territory. The first experiments were conducted over a period of three days in October, 1940, above Balsam Lake, about eighty kilometres northeast of Toronto.

The Royal Canadian Air Force provided a float plane and a box of sawdust. Different grades of sawdust were released over the lake at varying altitudes. The purpose was to find out if the sawdust was an effective means for spreading disease. Afterwards, Banting felt the experiments were a success. He believed the Allies had a job to do. The job was to kill as many "Huns" as possible, and to kill them without mercy. It was a matter of self-preservation.

Now that Banting and his team had found that sawdust was a suitable medium for spreading disease, they began to discuss which of the deadly microbes was best. Banting met with a group of scientists at his home, which overlooked the city of Toronto. They talked about using infectious diseases like plague and cholera to fight an enemy. The subject of building factories to produce diseases came up. The various ideas came to be known as Project M-1000, a secret except to the minister of defence and maybe the prime minister.

ꟹ

Through his membership in the NRC, Banting was involved in a number of military research projects, from radar to gas warfare to aircraft design. Towards the end of August, 1940, his diary even contains references to alpha, beta, and gamma rays, as well as uranium 235, which would be used in the manufacture of atom bombs. The scientific community had known since 1934 that radioactive uranium created energy when it was bombarded with neutrons. By 1939, scientists realized that the neutrons were splitting a uranium-235 nucleus in two, producing a chain reaction known as fission. The Americans began conducting their own research in Chicago and at Los Alamos, New Mexico, and five years later, in August, 1945, the United States dropped two atomic bombs on Japan, at Hiroshima and Nagasaki, ending the war.

Banting was comfortable with the NRC's participation in chemical warfare research. He believed that civilization was doomed if the Allies lost the war. But he was tired of bureaucracy. He wanted to be part of the action in Europe.

He didn't like going home to Rosedale Heights every evening after work when what he really wanted was to be a battalion medical officer, like he was in the First World War. His passion was healing, and there was no greater place to practise the healing arts than the theatre of war, surrounded by dying and wounded men. To be at home while the rest of the world was about to be dominated by the Nazis, who represented pure evil, was too much for Banting to bear. He wanted to be in Europe to fight the Nazis. He wanted to be part of the war and fight like a man.

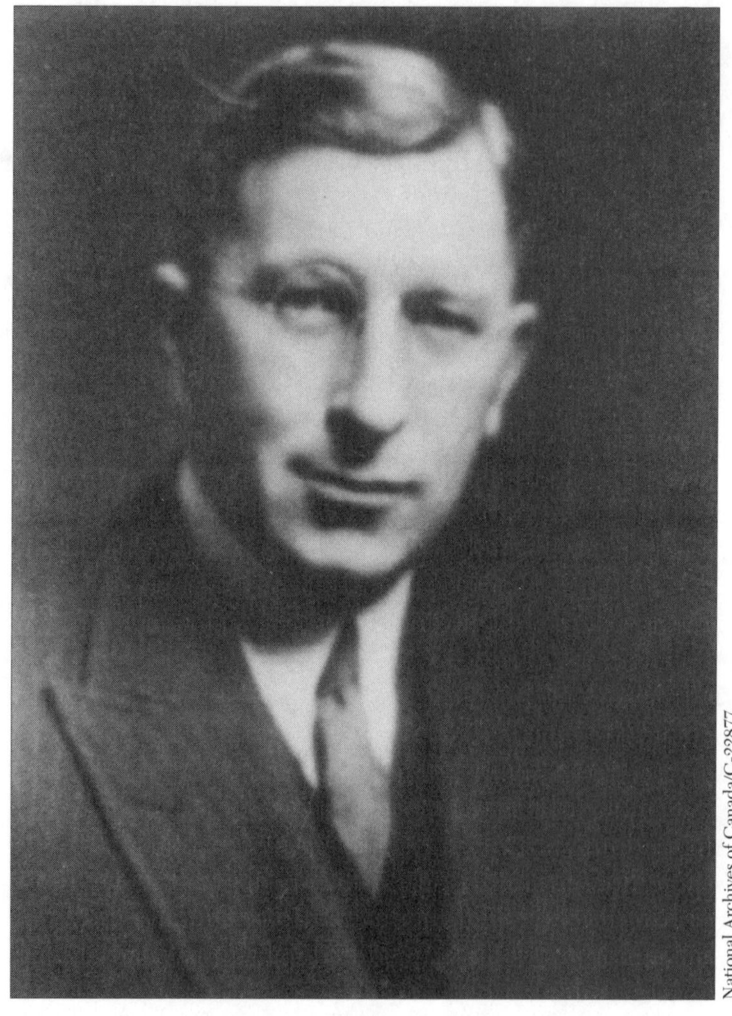

National Archives of Canada/C-22877.

Despite his faults and weaknesses, Banting was a great man who healed the sick and saved countless lives.

10

A Man Who Saved Lives

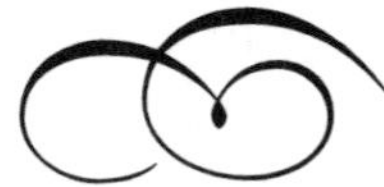

By November, 1940, Banting knew he wouldn't be going to England before the end of the year. His mother was eighty-six and bedridden. He had written to her every Sunday of his life. He visited her in Alliston on December 1, 1940. She died the next day.

The war began to consume him. Radio broadcasts from Europe reminded him of what was at stake. He had been donating any extra cash to the war effort. The Germans had entered Paris, and at Dunkirk over 300,000 British forces had to be evacuated.

He was busy with his NRC projects but still found time to visit Halifax and Quebec City to discuss local health problems. He suggested that post-graduate medical facilities be provided to those French Canadian medical students who were now unable to go to Paris because of the Nazi occupation.

Banting decided it was time for him to check on the status of military research in England and to strengthen Canada's role in aviation medicine projects with the British. He had already carried out decompression-sickness experiments in which he subjected himself to the disabling effects of high altitudes in a decompression chamber. He had flown in a fighter plane to study the effects on the human body of sudden changes in gravitational forces. He thought he might be able to get over to England and work near the front, where the fighting was, maybe help British pilots win the air war. He was sick and tired of being Sir Frederick Banting, the medical figurehead everyone wanted for their speeches and banquets. He despised bureaucratic life in Toronto. He began to plan to travel overseas. His son Bill was eleven. Banting promised the boy he'd give a good account of himself in England.

He considered getting passage to England on board a Canadian destroyer. But on January 31, 1941, at a cocktail party in Ottawa, he discovered that it might be possible to fly over to England on one of the twin-engined Hudson coastal reconnaissance bombers being ferried through Montreal to Britain.

Banting didn't want to stay in Canada any longer.

He could not forget the time, in the summer of 1940, when he walked over to the House of Commons to see the members of Parliament in action. He had to hobble because his leg had been badly burned in a gas warfare experiment for which he had volunteered. He had expected to see a debate on the war. Instead, he watched federal politicians talking about a grant to beautify the streets and sidewalks of Ottawa. The $100,000 being debated for municipal improvements was, at the time, more than the NRC had available to spend on non-military medical research across Canada. He felt the Canadian government was an easy mark for Hitler and the Nazis.

Now, at the end of January, there was the possibility that he could be part of the war sooner than he thought.

He was almost fifty years old. Every single day of his life had been filled with action or work. Work had been his salvation. Even when his medical practice was failing in London, back in 1920, he painted, and read, and planned. It now seemed likely that Hitler was going to take away his country, the only home he had ever known. He didn't want to attract attention to himself. He just wanted to get over to Europe and fight the Germans, even if it was only as a medical officer. Perhaps, he thought, his medical knowledge could be put to good use.

Authorization for a passage to England on one of the Hudson bombers was approved. Banting would have his chance to fight the Germans. He was thrilled.

He was in his lab when the call came on Saturday, February 15, 1941, ordering him to report to Montreal for the flight to England.

In Montreal, he was taken to a supply depot and outfitted for the flight. The only article of clothing he could not get was a pair of warm gloves.

It was a fairly new idea to fly the planes to England rather than shipping them by boat. Banting would be only the second passenger to cross the North Atlantic on one of these bombers.

The first shipment of Hudsons had reached the United Kingdom by sea in 1939, and it didn't take long for them to show their worth. A Hudson over Jutland had shot down the first German aircraft claimed by the Royal Air Force during the war, and the planes, which had a top speed of 370 kilometres per hour, were used over the Dunkirk beaches as dogfighters. They were made by Lockheed, an American civilian aviation company that also produced the P-38 Lightning for the war, a twin-engined fighter with a novel twin boom and central cockpit layout.

Waiting for the plane to leave, he met Bert Collip in his hotel room. Like Banting, Collip was a member of Canada's National Research Council.

Although Banting and Collip had fought twenty years ago in Toronto, over the discovery of insulin, they were friends now, and they reminisced about the insulin days. Collip, who would take over Banting's NRC duties while he was in England, wondered if he would be warm enough on his trans-Atlantic flight. They shared a cordial goodbye. Later in the day Collip left him a pair of sheepskin gloves at the hotel desk. Banting took the gloves with him on his way out.

The bomber left Saint-Hubert's Field outside Montreal at 9:50 a.m. on Monday, February 17. It was a skeleton craft with a ribbed interior, and none of the usual passenger-plane comforts.

The pilot was Joseph Mackey, a daredevil from Kansas City who was making his second flight ferrying the bombers to England. He got along well with Banting. He thought the doctor was a hard-fighting, hard-drinking man, the kind of guy you could trust. The radioman was Bill Snailham, and the navigator was William Bird.

Major Sir Frederick Banting was the only passenger. They had a smooth flight to the airbase at Gander, Newfoundland, 1400 kilometres away. There were reports of bad weather over Britain. At Gander they waited to take off with the crews of five other Hudsons. A blizzard settled in around the base. There wasn't much to do except talk, play cards, and drink whisky or coffee. Some of the men had colds, and Banting, always the physician, went out in the snow and brought back alcohol and medicine and hot water bottles.

It was tough to make a transatlantic flight in winter. Twenty-five Hudsons had made the trip so far. One had crashed on take-off. Another was forced to return to Gander because of mechanical problems. The civilian crews that were hired to do the ferrying had little experience flying these bombers on long-distance, winter flights. But Banting was told that the Hudsons were safe, and that you could fly the Atlantic, if you had to, on a single engine.

At 5:30 p.m. on February 20, Banting's plane roared down the lighted runway and took off for England.

The plane was over the Atlantic, about eighty kilometres northeast of Gander, when an oil cooler malfunctioned. Mackey shut down the starboard engine and was going to fly the plane with only one propeller when the oil supply to the port engine failed. Snailham, the radioman, asked Gander for bearings back to the airport. The dead Hudson shook violently and headed down in the dark.

Mackey jettisoned the fuel. "Throw out anything you can!" he shouted. "Anything! We have to maintain altitude!"

Banting made his way forward to the cockpit. He looked out the windscreen. It was dark, and snow was hitting the glass. He could feel the plane dropping. They were now over land, at about 2,000 feet.

"Put on your chute, Doc. You're gonna bail out. Be quick about it." Mackey turned to his radioman and his navigator. "You men do the same," he ordered.

Mackey used to barnstorm around the Midwest, skywriting and putting on shows for Kansas farmers. He was the kind of man Banting had always admired, a man with "guts." He was not going to abandon his plane. He was going to take it down, even if he died in the crash.

About twenty kilometres southwest of Musgrave Harbour, on Newfoundland's east coast, the bomber came down in the falling snow, sheared off the tops of some trees, and smashed into the woods just short of a frozen lake.

The impact knocked Mackey out. When he came to, he was still at the controls. The cabin was bathed in an eerie, silvery light from the flasks of sea markers that had burst on impact, showering the inside of the plane with aluminum powder. The others had not jumped. Mackey found the radioman and navigator both dead. Banting, semiconscious, lay on the floor of the cabin. He had smashed his head against the bulwark and broken his left arm. His left lung had been punctured by a fractured rib.

Mackey stumbled into the cabin and used parachute silk to make bandages and blankets for Banting. He moved the famed physician to a comfortable resting place. The aluminum powder had covered everything, even the bodies of the dead men, even Mackey and Banting, in an unearthly glow.

Mackey looked outside. It was still snowing. Everything was quiet. The only sound was the blizzard beating against the fuselage. Mackey had a sprained ankle. He limped outside to see where the plane had crashed. He had missed the frozen lake by only a couple of metres. The snowdrifts were almost as tall as a man. He came back inside and turned off all the lights in the plane but one. He attended to Banting, who was slipping in and out of consciousness. Delirious, Banting began dictating ideas and thoughts to the pilot, who pretended to write them down, so as not to upset him. But it was impossible to understand his urgent, scientific riddles. Banting would lie back, rest, then sit up again. The wind howled all night.

In the morning, Mackey was weak and in shock. Despite his injured ankle, the pilot decided to get help. He built crude snowshoes out of friction tape and the pieces of a wooden map board.

"Doc, I'm going to get us out of here."

Banting opened his eyes and began to talk.

"You know physicians give strange medicines to their patients... two injections of 10 cc each...it is a universal pill, good against all the diseases that pilgrims are incident to...pancreatic lythiasis...."

"I can't understand you."

"...if man will but use this physic as he should, it will make him live forever...glycosuria and ketonuria have almost disappeared...from this world to that which is to come...the moon...is it snowing outside?"

"Snowing lightly, Doc. The worst is over."

"It's snowing in Saint-Fidèle."

"Try to rest, pal. I'm going to get help."

Banting closed his eyes. He seemed to be asleep. Covering Banting with coats, the pilot left the plane. Walking through the deep snow made him tired. He thought he could see houses, and lighted windows, but when he got closer they were only snow-covered trees and rocks. It took him all day to cover three kilometres. When he returned that night, he found Banting. The great man had awakened in the cabin and managed to climb outside. He fell forward into the snow and died, not five metres from the plane.

Search planes were not able to take off until the 21st, the day Banting died. They could not find the downed plane. Snow had been falling since the crash and all but covered the fuselage. Rescuers were still looking Sunday, February 23, when the world was informed that Sir Frederick Banting was missing on a flight to England.

Mackey ate frozen oranges and rations. He slept in the cold huddled under coats, and planned another journey on makeshift snowshoes. He tried lighting signal fires with gasoline from the plane. But the twigs were too frozen to burn, and the search planes passed overhead.

On Monday, February 24, he broke one of the sea flasks and scattered aluminum dust around the plane. The signal, a black streak in the snow, was seen by a passing Hudson. Planes appeared and began to drop provisions. Realizing the rescuers didn't know what had happened to the others, Mackey tramped words in the snow: THREE DEAD – JOE. One of the planes dropped a message to rabbit trappers who were nearby, letting them know about the plane. The trappers found Mackey and took him back to Musgrave Harbour.

A search party from the village later retrieved the dead bodies. Bird and Snailham were buried in Halifax. Mackey was taken to Montreal. He sold the exclusive rights of Banting's last flight to the *Toronto Star*, and gave the money to Snailham's three children, who were left without parents.

Despite Mackey's published account, rumours persisted. Was Banting carrying top-secret intelligence for the British? Did Nazi agents in North America sabotage the plane? The rumours were never confirmed. Banting wanted to go to England for one reason. He wanted to get away from Toronto and be a man again. He wanted to fight in the war.

A private service for Banting was held in Toronto on Monday, March 3. The body was moved to the University of Toronto's Convocation Hall, where it lay in state the next morning. The flag-draped casket was placed on a gun carriage, and the funeral procession and military escort made its way through the streets of

Toronto, accompanied by an RCAF pipe band that played the funeral march.

Sir Frederick Grant Banting was buried in Mount Pleasant Cemetery. He was only forty-nine years old when he died. He was dressed, not in the rough clothes of a farmer, but in the uniform of a major in the Canadian Army. Banting, who had been a decorated war hero in the First World War, was proud of his military service, but he was equally proud of being a farmer's son. To the end of his life, he remained an unpolished man who was also a hero. For thousands of years, diabetes had been a mystery. The disease perplexed physicians; even the name "diabetes" frightened people. Banting fought the medical establishment, and the belief that a treatment would never be found, and won. Countless children and young people throughout the world owed him their lives, and their families would never forget that.

Banting had to wrestle his own personal demons, but he believed in himself and the power of his imagination. His idea for insulin, an idea that forever changed the world, came to him on a sleepless night. As a researcher, his primary method was trial-and-error. He compared scientific work to the work of Sherlock Holmes, a fictional character in detective novels who solved mysteries by combining intense preparation with intuition.

In some ways, Banting was a throwback to the time of seventeenth-century physicist Isaac Newton, when science was still related to art, and to alchemy, a medieval chemical science and philosophy that aimed at discovering the principle behind all life and a universal cure for all disease. To Banting, scientists and artists had much in common. Scientific achievement, like great art, was the result of intuition and hard work. Later, when he began to pursue his passion for painting, he came to believe that scientists, like artists, were rebels who worked on the fringes of society.

Banting loved to explore the unknown, whether it was a snowy night in rural Quebec, or the frontiers of medicine. He liked to paint, sleep under the stars, and read detective stories. Most of all, he liked being a doctor. Money and fame were not important to him, healing was. At the end of the day, all he wanted to know was that he had brought health to his patients.

When he was a boy on the farm near Alliston, he used to stare at the tiny glass door on the kitchen clock with the painted palm trees and faded moon. The shy boy who couldn't spell would never have imagined, though, that one day an idea he scribbled down in the middle of the night would bring children back from the brink of death. Sitting there, staring at the clock, he could not have imagined that schools would be named after him, or that books would be written about him, or, impossibly, that one of the craters on the moon, named after the great scientists of history, would one day be named after him, in honour of what he had done.

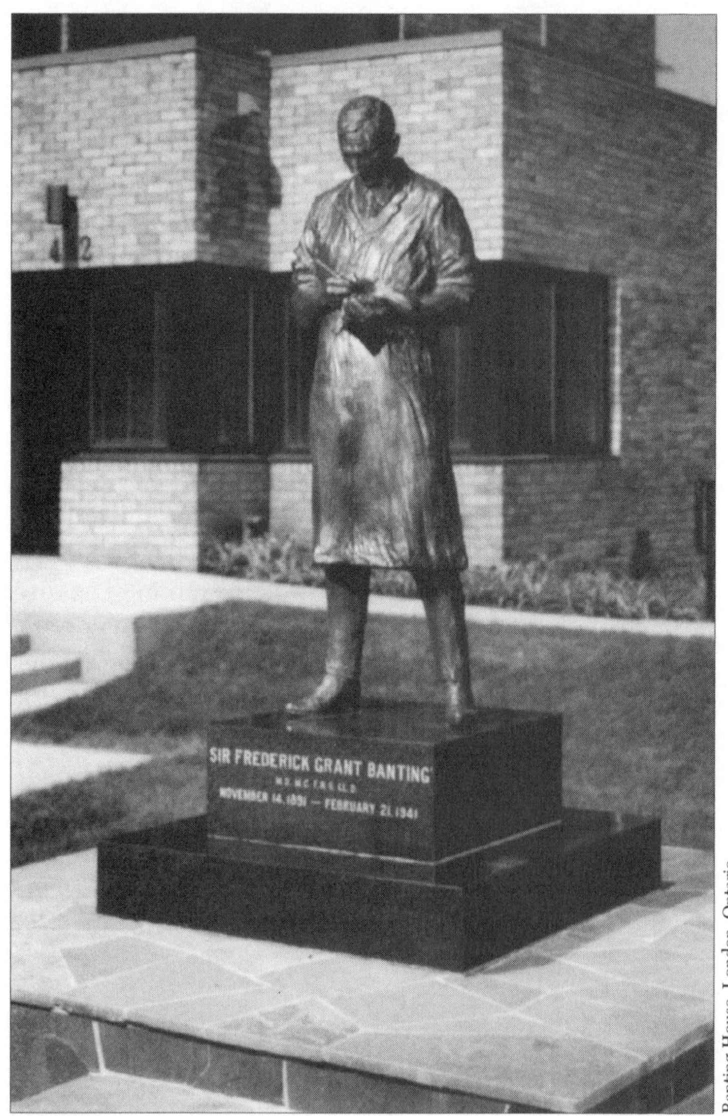

Banting House, London, Ontario.

This statue of Banting in London, Ontario, commemorates his life-saving work.

Chronology of Frederick Banting (1891-1941)

Compiled by Lynne Bowen

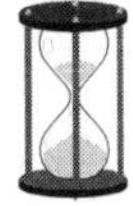

BANTING AND HIS TIMES

CANADA AND THE WORLD

1678
English religious writer John Bunyan publishes *Pilgrim's Progress*.

1839
The College of Physicians and Surgeons of Upper Canada is incorporated.

1840
English novelist Charles Dickens publishes *The Old Curiosity Shop*, in installments.

1847
The College of Physicians and Surgeons of Lower Canada is created; one of its founders, Dr. Edward Dagge Worthington, pioneers the use of general anesthesia in Canada in this year.

BANTING AND HIS TIMES

1854
Banting's mother, Margaret, is born.

CANADA AND THE WORLD

1867
In Scotland, Joseph Lister initiates antiseptic surgery by using carbolic acid on a wound.

In the midst of a turbulent period in Canadian medicine, the Canadian Medical Association is formed.

1869
Dr. Archibald Malloch, having studied with Lister in Glasgow, attempts to convince other Canadian doctors of the value of antiseptic surgery.

1874
The Ontario Agricultural College is founded in Guelph.

1875
The Theosophical Society is founded in New York by Helena Petrova Blavatsky.

1876
John James Rickard Macleod, future co-discoverer of insulin, is born at Cluny, Scotland.

In Britain, the Cruelty to Animals Act imposes a system of licensing and inspection on British researchers – a clear victory for the anti-vivisectionists.

Banting and His Times	**Canada and the World**

1878
The Western University of London, later the University of Western Ontario, is founded.

Alexander Young (A.Y.) Jackson, future Canadian painter, writer and nationalist, is born in Montreal.

1884
In Canada, different groups of Methodists unite to form one Methodist Church.

1887
The Faculty of Medicine at the University of Toronto (U of T) is restored after having been abolished in the 1850s.

Arthur Conan Doyle, an English doctor who began writing to pass the time while waiting for patients who never came, publishes the first Sherlock Holmes story, "A Study in Scarlet," in *Beeton's Christmas Annual*.

1889
German scientists Von Mehring and Minkowski prove that the pancreas secretes a substance that appears to have a connection with diabetes mellitus.

c.1890
Most Canadian surgeons have begun to use sterile methods when they operate.

BANTING AND HIS TIMES

1891
Frederick Grant Banting, the sixth child of William and Margaret Banting, is born on November 14 in their farmhouse near Alliston, Ontario.

CANADA AND THE WORLD

1891
The first Canadian branch of the Theosophical Society is formed in Toronto.

Arthur Conan Doyle publishes "The Adventures of Sherlock Holmes" in *Strand* magazine.

1892
Canada's Dr. William Osler publishes his authoritative textbook *The Principles and Practice of Medicine*.

1899
Charles Herbert Best, future co-discoverer of insulin, is born at West Pembroke, Maine.

The Boer War begins in South Africa; Canada sends troops to support Britain; the war divides Canadians along French and English lines.

1901
Prince Edward Island becomes the first Canadian province to enact Prohibition.

George Mercer Dawson, Canadian geologist, dies in Ottawa.

1902
Arthur Conan Doyle publishes *The Hound of the Baskervilles*; he is knighted for his work in a field hospital during the Boer War, which has just ended.

Banting and His Times	**Canada and the World**
1903 Banting is forced to wear his sister's hand-me-down boots to school; he wins a fight with a bully; his mother buys him boy's boots.	**1903** Sir William Osler opens the medical building at the University of Toronto. Dr. J.J.R. Macleod emigrates from Scotland to Cleveland, Ohio.
	1904 Russian physiologist Ivan Petrovich Pavlov is awarded the Nobel Prize for his experiments on conditioned reflexes of the nervous system.
	1905 Dr. William Osler becomes Regius professor of medicine at Oxford University in England.
	1908 The Arts and Letters Club of Toronto is founded.
1910 Banting has grown tall and has an athletic build; having chosen to study medicine, he enrolls in Victoria College at U of T.	
1911 Banting meets Edith Roach, daughter of a Methodist minister.	**1911** Dr. William Osler is made a baronet. Britain's King Edward VII dies and is succeeded by his son, George V.
1912 Banting spends the spring and summer helping his father on the	**1912** The S.S. *Titanic* sinks.

Banting and His Times

farm; although he must make up failed German and French courses, he is allowed to enter medical school.

1914
Banting tries to enlist in the Canadian Army, but is rejected twice because of poor eyesight.

1915
The army finally having accepted him, Banting spends the summer in a training camp in Niagara Falls then returns to complete his fourth year of medical school.

1916
Banting completes his fifth year of medical school in a special accelerated summer session; he receives his Bachelor of Medicine degree in December; Norman Bethune is a classmate.

Canada and the World

1913
J.J.R. Macleod publishes a book on diabetes, which states that the internal secretion of the pancreas can never be isolated.

Aboriginal poet E. Pauline Johnson dies in Vancouver.

1914
Britain declares war on Germany; Canada is automatically at war; young Canadians flock to join the army.

Connaught Laboratories Limited, a producer of biological products including vaccines, is established in the Department of Hygiene at U of T.

1915
At the Second Battle of Ypres in Belgium, the Germans use chlorine gas for the first time; two days later, on April 24, the First Canadian Division is gassed.

1916
In Canada, the National Research Council (NRC) is founded to fund research committees for special needs and offer university science fellowships.

BANTING AND HIS TIMES

1917
In March, Banting sails from Halifax to England where he is posted to a hospital for soldiers maimed or blinded by poison gas.

1918
Banting is transferred to a Canadian hospital in France and then to a field ambulance unit in the Amiens-Arras sector; in August he is posted to the front lines as medical officer to the 44th Battalion, 4th Canadian Division; the unit joins the battle around Cambrai, where 40,000 men will die; Banting crosses open territory to rescue another medical officer; in September he is wounded in the right arm, and though seriously injured, defies orders and stays to treat the other wounded.

Banting is awarded the Military Cross and is sent to England; he spends nine weeks in hospital and refuses to allow doctors to amputate his arm; he leaves hospital in December three weeks after the war ends; the war has destroyed his belief in God.

CANADA AND THE WORLD

1917
On December 6, at 8:45 a.m., two ships collide in Halifax harbour, causing the greatest manmade explosion yet.

Canadian painter Tom Thomson drowns mysteriously in Canoe Lake, Algonquin Park.

The October (Bolshevik) Revolution in Russia deposes the monarchy.

1918
World War One (WWI) ends; over eight million have died and twenty-one million have been wounded.

In Canada, all female citizens (except status Indians) are eligible to vote in federal elections,

J.J.R. Macleod becomes professor of physiology at U of T.

In Russia, the Bolsheviks execute ex-Czar Nicholas II and his entire family.

A worldwide influenza epidemic kills twenty-two million people in two years.

BANTING AND HIS TIMES

1919
In March, Banting returns to Canada; he is posted to the Christie Street Hospital in Toronto where he does orthopedic work on wounded and crippled soldiers.

In summer he is discharged from the army; he becomes a senior house surgeon at the Hospital for Sick Children; he has no money and his fiancée, Edith, wants to get married.

1920
Banting moves to London, Ontario; he sets up a practice but has few patients; he sketches to pass the time; he teaches himself to paint and tries unsuccessfully to sell his work.

In the early hours of October 31, Banting reads an article by Dr. Moses Barron on pancreatic lithiasis; at 2:00 a.m., he scribbles twenty-five words in his notebook which are the germ of an idea to treat diabetes mellitus; a week later he visits Dr. J.J.R. Macleod at U of T and asks to be allowed to test his idea; Macleod suggests he try his experiment the following summer.

1921
Unsure of himself, Banting applies for a job in the North; when the job falls through he decides to go ahead with his experiment but just for the summer.

CANADA AND THE WORLD

1919
In Canada, Prohibition is repealed in Quebec; Sir William Osler dies; women are allowed to be candidates in federal elections.

The Treaty of Versailles sets the terms for post-WWI peace.

1920
Prohibition is enacted in the United States (U.S.); Prohibition is repealed in British Columbia (B.C.)

In Canada, painters Franklin Carmichael, Lawren Harris, A.Y. Jackson, Franz Johnston, Arthur Lismer, J.E.H. MacDonald and F.H. Varley form the Group of Seven; they become closely associated with the Theosophical Society.

Adolf Hitler, an obscure Austrian politician, announces his 25-point program in Munich.

1921
The Communist Party of Canada is founded as a secret organization in Guelph, Ontario.

Banting and His Times

In May, Macleod sets Banting up in a small U of T laboratory; he assigns him a student research assistant named Charley Best, who has won the job over Clark Noble on the toss of a coin; Banting and Best begin to operate on laboratory dogs and learn by making many mistakes. They suffer through the hot summer and work around the clock.

On August 9, Banting writes to Macleod, who is in Scotland, to tell him that he and Best have produced "isletin," an extract that reduces blood and urinary sugar in diabetic dogs; a collie named Number 92 lives for several days until they run out of isletin.

In September, Banting sells his house in London; Macleod returns from Scotland, and although unsympathetic to Banting's demands for better working conditions, finally agrees to pay him and Best for their work and provide a lab assistant.

Banting and Best begin to work with pancreases from calf fetuses; in November Banting demonstrates the safety of the extract by injecting himself subcutaneously; he is soon able to produce extract from whole beef pancreases.

In December, University of Alberta biochemist, James Bertram (Bert) Collip, joins the

Canada and the World

Agnes Macphail becomes the first woman to be elected to the Canadian Parliament.

William Lyon Mackenzie King becomes prime minister of Canada.

Banting and His Times

research team; he discovers that the extract will restore the liver's ability to store glycogen; Banting's classmate, Joe Gilchrist, a diabetic, takes isletin orally, but it has no effect; Banting presents his results to the American Physiological Society conference at Yale University; he begins to suspect Collip and Macleod of stealing his work.

1922
On January 11, Leonard Thompson becomes the first human diabetic to have isletin injected into his body; impurities in the extract cause an abscess to develop.

On January 16, Collip succeeds in purifying the extract; insulin is precipitated out; seven days later, Thompson revives immediately after receiving an injection of the purified extract; when Collip refuses to reveal his process, Banting attacks him physically; Macleod makes Collip, Banting and Best agree not to patent the extract individually.

On May 3, Macleod presents a paper to the Association of American physicians in Washington, D.C.; he summarizes the work and calls the extract "insulin"; Banting is in Toronto "celebrating" by himself.

As diabetics from all over North America converge on Toronto,

Canada and the World

1922
The Union of Soviet Socialist Republics (U.S.S.R.) is formed from the former Russian empire.

Benito Mussolini and his Italian fascists march on Rome and form the government.

The Communist Party of Canada changes its name to the Workers' Party and begins to work in the open.

Banting and His Times	**Canada and the World**
Collip is unable to repeat his purifying process; Banting, Best, and Macleod try to rediscover the extract without success; a young girl dies when they can produce no more insulin; the pressure causes Banting to drink heavily until Best persuades him to carry on.	
Two months later, Banting and Best have produced useable insulin; they work with patients from the Christie Street Military Hospital, which has opened a diabetic clinic; Banting gives a batch of insulin to American Dr. John Williams to treat the son of a vice-president of Eastman-Kodak.	
U of T continues to refuse an appointment to Banting, who is regarded as wild, impulsive, and temperamental.	
Banting, Macleod, Best, and Collip accept a proposal from Eli Lilly and Company to collaborate; although Best is in charge of insulin production at Connaught Lab, the poor equipment affects the quality of the insulin being produced; when the U of T board of governors drags its feet, Banting receives help from a wealthy American.	
In August, American doctors Elliott Joslin and Frederick Allen begin clinical trials on their diabetic patients; the diabetic clinic at Toronto General Hospital opens	

Banting and His Times

with Banting as attending physician; the Connaught Lab is now producing potent insulin using new equipment purchased with American money.

Banting begins to treat Elizabeth Hughes; three months later, in November, her American doctors, Joslin and Allen, visit Toronto and are astounded at how she has improved.

1923
Nominations for the Nobel Prize in Physiology or Medicine have been arriving in Stockholm, Sweden, since December 1922; Banting and Macleod are each nominated separately; August Krogh, a Danish physiologist and Nobel Laureate nominates them as a team.

In the summer, Banting sails for England on board the *Empress of France*; on July 18, he is presented to King George V; he delivers several speeches on his work; he returns to Canada and hides unsuccessfully from reporters.

The Ontario government establishes the Banting and Best Chair of Medical Research at U of T; Banting is named permanent Professor of Medical Research; the House of Commons grants him a lifetime annuity of $7,500.

Canada and the World

1923
In Canada, U of T's Dr. W.E. Brown establishes the value of ethylene as a general anesthetic.

Hitler's "Beer Hall Putsch" fails in Munich, Germany.

BANTING AND HIS TIMES

Banting opens the Canadian National Exhibition in Toronto on August 25; medals with his likeness on one side are awarded to achievers; he is finally able to return to work in the fall.

When Banting reads in the newspaper in October that he and Macleod have been awarded the Nobel Prize, he is furious because Best has been left out.

Banting and Macleod announce that they will share the prize with Best and Collip.

Although Banting speaks well of Macleod when they are given honorary Doctor of Science degrees at U of T, he is still bitter.

1924
In May, Banting and Edith Roach sign an agreement breaking off their engagement; he courts Marion Robertson, an X-ray technician from Elora, Ontario; they marry quietly on June 4.

Banting's efforts to find the "elixir of life" by isolating antitoxins in the adrenal cortex are unsuccessful.

Banting receives an honorary degree from Yale University; he and Marion honeymoon in the Caribbean for two months; he attends conferences, presents

CANADA AND THE WORLD

1924
Vladimir Ilyich Lenin, first premier of the U.S.S.R., dies; the name of St. Petersburg is changed to Leningrad; Josef Stalin struggles with Leon Trotsky for power.

BANTING AND HIS TIMES

papers, and tours medical facilities while Marion socializes.

On their return in September, the Bantings move into a grand house; their first house guest is Lord Dawson of Penn, physician to King George V.

1925
In January, Banting contributes two small paintings to an exhibit of the work of U of T staff and students; Lawren Harris nominates Banting for membership in the Arts and Letters Club.

In August the Bantings sail for Europe on the *Empress of Scotland* in great luxury; they go to Stockholm for Banting's Nobel address; he is touched by the gratitude of Swedish diabetics.

1926
While returning by train from giving a speech in Victoria, B.C., Banting leaves the train to visit a severely ill diabetic living in a remote settlement in the mountains.

1927
Wishing to be like Arthur Conan Doyle, Banting creates a fictional detective named Silas Eagles; he submits a story to the International Magazine Company but it is rejected.

CANADA AND THE WORLD

1925
The United Church of Canada is formed by a merger of the Congregationalist and Methodist Churches and a majority of Presbyterians.

In Germany, Hitler publishes volume I of *Mein Kampf*.

1927
B.C. painter Emily Carr meets the Group of Seven; their encouragement stimulates her art and helps her achieve maturity in her painting.

BANTING AND HIS TIMES

In March, Group of Seven painter A.Y. Jackson invites Banting on a sketching trip to St. Jean Port Jolie in Quebec; Banting travels under the alias, "Frederick Grant."

In the summer, Banting serves as a volunteer medical officer on the steamer *Beothic* as she resupplies settlements and Royal Canadian Mounted Police (RCMP) posts in the Eastern Arctic; A.Y. Jackson goes too; the two men paint together on the deck of the ship; bad weather keeps them at Beechey Island, where Sir John Franklin and his men spent their last winter in 1845-46.

Living conditions of the Inuit shock Banting; he allows an interview with the *Toronto Star*'s Roy Greenaway, whose article the next day appears under the headline, "Banting Regrets Hudson Bay Use of Eskimo"; in the charges and countercharges that follow, Banting feels betrayed by the press again; he submits two reports to the Department of the Interior on the health of the Inuit.

CANADA AND THE WORLD

Charles Lindbergh flies his monoplane nonstop from New York to Paris, the first solo transatlantic flight.

1928

Banting begins a five-year-long experiment in which he transplants tumour-causing material into Plymouth Rock chickens in the hope that he can find a vaccine to fight cancer.

1928

The Communist Party of Canada is ordered by the Third International of the Communist Party to start trade unions; they set up the Workers' Unity League to coordinate union activities.

BANTING AND HIS TIMES

Although the Bantings give the appearance of marital happiness in public, they are growing apart; Banting is drinking and smoking excessively.

Banting and A.Y. Jackson go to Great Slave Lake to explore and sketch.

1929
In an unsuccessful effort to salvage their marriage, the Bantings have a son, William; a divorce being difficult to obtain, he proposes that they "live outside the boundaries of marriage."

Banting meets Blodwen Davies, a freelance writer who is researching the death of painter Tom Thomson; Blodwen persuades him to attend meetings of the Theosophical Society.

Banting becomes chairman of a research program studying silicosis.

1930
Banting and A.Y. Jackson go to Saint-Fidèle, Quebec to sketch, snowshoe, and lunch in the outdoors.

1931
Marion Banting meets Donat M. LeBourdais, a broadcaster and

CANADA AND THE WORLD

Josef Stalin becomes leader of the U.S.S.R.

In Britain, Alexander Fleming discovers penicillin and suggests possibilities for the treatment of disease.

1929
Charles Best succeeds J.J.R. Macleod as professor of physiology at U of T; Macleod returns to Scotland.

On October 28, Black Friday, the American stock exchange collapses; the ten-year-long Great Depression begins.

The Kellogg-Briand Pact outlawing war is signed by sixty-five countries.

1930
In Canada, all provinces except Prince Edward Island have repealed Prohibition; the Conservatives under R.B. Bennett win the federal election.

Sir Arthur Conan Doyle dies.

1931
The divorce rate in Canada is very low; divorce actions in Ontario are

Banting and His Times

employee of the Canadian National Committee on Mental Hygiene.

1932
In order to "prove" adultery and give grounds for divorce under Canada's antiquated laws, Banting and two detectives break in on Marion and Donat. Banting moves out of his home the next day; a divorce is granted quietly on April 25, but the press publishes a front-page account; one week before the divorce is to become final, Marion's father and Donat file motions of intervention; headlines declare that Banting is cruel to Marion. The divorce goes ahead as planned; Marion gets custody of their son, who visits his father on weekends at his apartment near the university.

1933
Banting goes to Europe for two months; he attends the International Cancer Congress in Madrid, goes to a bullfight, and paints.

1934
Banting is made Knight Commander of the Civil Division of the Order of the British Empire; Sir Frederick Banting, K.B.E. is uncomfortable with his title but it proves he has not been disgraced by his divorce.

Canada and the World

transferred from federal jurisdiction to the Supreme Court of Ontario.

1932
The Nazi Party wins a majority in the German Reichstag elections.

1933
Adolf Hitler is appointed German chancellor.

1934
Dr. Elliott Joslin addresses the opening ceremonies of new Eli Lilly research laboratories and likens the discovery of insulin to the Bible story about Ezekiel and the army of the slain who come back to life.

Banting and His Times	**Canada and the World**
1935 Banting sails to England to be inducted into the Royal Society of London; he boards the steamship *Smolny* to sail to Leningrad to attend the Fifteenth International Physiological Congress; he visits Ivan Pavlov; he is impressed by a militaristic parade of athletes but as he tours the country notices the discrepancy between propaganda and reality; forced by circumstance to leave the U.S.S.R. by slow train, he travels through Germany where swastika flags are flying everywhere. Despite the realities he witnessed in the U.S.S.R., Banting begins calling himself a communist and referring to his friends as "comrade," but he soon tires of it and never joins the Communist Party	**1935** Canadian doctor Norman Bethune attends the Fifteenth International Physiological Congress in Leningrad. In Canada, the On to Ottawa Trek of unemployed men is stopped in Regina by the RCMP; William Lyon Mackenzie King succeeds R.B. Bennett as prime minister and appoints Vincent Massey as High Commissioner to Great Britain; Tommy Douglas, future father of Canadian medicare, is among five members of the Co-operative Commonwealth Federation (CCF) to be elected to the House of Commons; General Andrew McNaughton becomes president of the National Research Council. J.J.R. Macleod dies in Scotland. In Germany, the Nazis repudiate the Treaty of Versailles.
1936 Banting moves to a house overlooking Toronto, where he grows roses and his son, Bill, visits him frequently.	**1936** General Franco leads a fascist rebellion against the Spanish Republic; Norman Bethune goes to Spain and establishes the Canadian Blood Transfusion Service.
1937 In March, Banting and Jackson go on a sketching trip to Saint-Tite-des-Cap, Quebec.	**1937** Spanish rebels take Malaga and destroy Guernica; Japan invades China; Italy joins the Anti-Comintern pact and withdraws from the League of Nations.

Banting and His Times / **Canada and the World**

Alarmed by the possibility of war in Europe, Banting immerses himself in military research and top-secret bacterial warfare projects and prepares a confidential memo on germ warfare for General McNaughton of the NRC.

He meets twenty-five-year-old Henrietta Ball, a U of T graduate student; they begin a tumultuous relationship; when she goes to England he follows her.

1938

Banting, as chairman of the NRC's Associate Committee on Medical Research, tours Canadian universities and public health laboratories; he pleads for more government money so young scientists will stay in Canada.

1938

Hitler marches into Austria and takes control; Germany mobilizes; France calls up reservists; U.S. recalls its ambassador to Germany.

1939

Banting has so many responsibilities and distractions, he barely has time for his lab work; he is drinking and smoking heavily.

Banting marries Henrietta in June making her Lady Banting; they honeymoon on Georgian Bay.

In September, Banting re-enlists in the Royal Canadian Medical Corps as a pathologist; although he wants to see action, he is instead ordered to continue his research with the NRC; he is promoted to major; he goes to England to visit the Ministry of Supply's Chemical

1939

In September, Germany invades Poland; Britain declares war on Germany thus beginning World War II (WWII); Canada declares war.

The first shipment of Hudson reconnaissance bombers reaches England by sea from the American civil aviation company, Lockheed.

Banting and His Times	**Canada and the World**
Defence Experimental Station; he argues that the Allies should use bacterial warfare before the Germans do.	
1940 Banting sails for home in January, having enlisted the help of his friend Vincent Massey, the High Commissioner to London, to propose a bacterial warfare research centre to the British.	**1940** Between May 27 and June 2, over 300,000 British and Canadian troops, trapped by the German advance into France, are evacuated from Dunkirk, a French port on the English Channel.
In June, Banting begins to explore ways to spread biological agents; in July he meets with a group of bacteriologists and virologists at U of T; the first experiments using sawdust are conducted successfully in October above Balsam Lake, northeast of Toronto; meetings continue at Banting's house for the top-secret Project M-1000.	The Communist Party of Canada is banned by the War Measures Act and is re-formed as the Labour-Progressive Party. In the Canadian federal election, John Diefenbaker, future Canadian prime minister, is elected to the House of Commons for the first time.
Banting burns his leg badly in a warfare experiment, one of many he has conducted.	Winston Churchill becomes prime minister of Great Britain.
By August, Banting is interested in alpha, beta, and gamma rays, and uranium 235 (used in atomic bombs).	
In December, Banting's mother, Margaret, dies in Alliston.	
1941 Tired of being a medical figurehead, Banting is anxious to join the fight against Germany; in February he receives orders to	**1941** On December 7, Japanese planes attack Pearl Harbor, a U.S. naval base in Hawaii. The U.S. enters the war.

Banting and His Times

report to Montreal for a flight to Britain on a Hudson coastal reconnaissance bomber; while waiting for the plane he meets Bert Collip, who gives him a pair of winter gloves; the plane leaves Montreal on February 17 and flies to Gander, Newfoundland, where it must wait out a blizzard.

Banting's plane takes off for Britain on February 20; a malfunction causes the pilot to turn back but the plane crashes twenty kilometres southwest of Musgrave Harbour, Newfoundland; Banting and the pilot survive the crash but Banting dies the next day while the pilot goes for help.

On February 23 the world learns that Banting is missing; searchers find the plane on February 24; the pilot sells his story to the *Toronto Star*.

A private funeral service is held in Toronto on March 3 for Banting; the body lies in state in U of T's Convocation Hall on March 4, then the casket rides through the streets of Toronto on a gun carriage, a Royal Canadian Air Force pipe band playing the funeral march; Banting is buried in Mount Pleasant cemetery.

Canada and the World

The British government establishes a microbiological research station at Porton.

1942

Canadian Dr. Harold Griffith advances the science of anesthesia by using curare.

Banting and His Times | **Canada and the World**

The murder of Jews in German-held concentration camps begins.

Italian-born U.S. physicist Enrico Fermi produces the first controlled nuclear chain reaction.

1945
The first atomic bomb is detonated near Alamogordo, New Mexico in July; the U.S. drops atomic bombs on Japan in August, thus ending WWII.

1965
James Bertram Collip, who has become one of Canada's leading endocrinologists, dies in London, Ontario.

1967
Charles Best retires from U of T after a productive research career.

1978
Charles Best dies in Toronto.

Sources Consulted

BLISS, Michael. *The Discovery of Insulin*. Toronto: McClelland and Stewart, 1982, and University of Toronto Press, 2000.

BLISS, Michael. *Banting: A Biography*. Toronto: McClelland and Stewart, 1984.

BUNYAN, John. *The Pilgrim's Progress*. London: Ward, Lock & Co., Limited, 1910.

DICKENS, Charles. *The Old Curiosity Shop and Master Humphrey's Clock*. London: MacMillan and Co., Limited, 1927.

GROVE, Noel, ed. *Atlas of World History*. Washington, D.C.: National Geographic Society, 1997.

HARRIS, Seale. *Banting's Miracle: The Story of the Discoverer of Insulin*. Toronto: J.M. Dent & Sons (Canada) Limited, 1946.

HILL, Christopher. *A Tinker and a Poor Man: John Bunyan and his Church, 1628-1688*. New York: Alfred A. Knopf, Inc., 1988.

HOLMES, Tony. *Jane's Pocket Guide of Fighters of World War II*. New York: HarperCollins Publishers, 1999.

JACK, Donald. *Rogues, Rebels, and Geniuses: The Story of Canadian Medicine*. Toronto: Doubleday Canada Limited, 1981.

JACKSON, A.Y. *Banting As An Artist*. Toronto: The Ryerson Press, 1943.

KENWARD, Lucy, ed. *Canvas of War: Painting the Canadian Experience, 1914 to 1945*. Toronto: Douglas and McIntyre, Ltd., with the Canadian War Museum and the Canadian Museum of Civilization, 2000.

MASSEY, the Rt. Hon. Vincent and FERGUSON, George; LEBEL, Maurice; LAMB, W. Kaye; and NEATBY, Hilda. *Great Canadians: A Century of Achievement*. Toronto: The Canadian Centennial Publishing Company, 1965.

MITCHINSON, Wendy and MCGINNIS, Janice Dickin. *Essays in the History of Canadian Medicine*. Toronto: McClelland and Stewart, 1988. "J.B. Collip: A Forgotten Member of the Insulin Team," by Michael Bliss.

MURRAY, Joan. *Canadian Art in the Twentieth Century*. Toronto: Dundura Press, 1999.

NEWLANDS, Anne, ed. *Canadian Art From the Beginnings to 2000*. Willowdale: Firefly Books, 2000.

ORWELL, George. *1984*. New York: Signet Books (The New American Library), 1952.

PRATT, Viola Whitney. *Canadian Portraits* (Osler, Banting, Penfield): Famous Doctors. Toronto: Clarke, Irwin and Company Limited, 1956.

ROWLAND, John. *The Insulin Man: The Story of Sir Frederick Banting*. New York: Roy Publishers,Inc., 1965.

SHARPE, Mike. *Aircraft of World War II*. London: Brown Partworks Limited, 2000.

SHAW, Margaret Mason. *He Conquered Death: The Story of Frederick Grant Banting*. Toronto: The Macmillan Company of Canada Limited, 1946.

STALLINGS, Laurence, ed. *The First World War: A Photographic History*. New York: Simon and Schuster, 1933.

STEVENSON, Lloyd. *Sir Frederick Banting*. Toronto: The Ryerson Press, 1946

STRODE, Hudson. *The Pageant of Cuba*. New York: Random House, 1936.

SUCHLICKI, Jaime. *Cuba: From Columbus to Castro*. New York: Charles Scribner's Sons, 1974.

WALKER, Evans and MORA, Gilles. *Walker Evans Havana 1933*. London: Thames and Hudson Ltd., 1989.

WRENSHALL, G.A., HETENYI, G., FEASBY, W.R. *The Story of Insulin: Forty Years of Success Against Diabetes*. Printed in Great Britain for Max Reinhardt (Canada) Ltd., Toronto, by the Stellar Press, Ltd., Barnet, England, 1962.

Index

Printed in June 2001
at AGMV/Marquis,
Cap-Saint-Ignace (Québec).